End of Life Care in Neurological Disease

David Oliver
Editor

End of Life Care in Neurological Disease

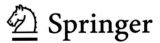 Springer

Editor
David Oliver BSc FRCP FRCGP
Wisdom Hospice
Rochester
Kent
UK

ISBN 978-0-85729-681-8   ISBN 978-0-85729-682-5   (eBook)
DOI 10.1007/978-0-85729-682-5
Springer London Heidelberg New York Dordrecht

Library of Congress Control Number: 2012952726

Printed on acid-free paper

Springer is part of Springer Science+Business Media (www.springer.com)

Foreword

In 2010, a group of health and social care professionals, together with representative patient organisations, met to consider the needs of people with progressive neurological disease. The meeting was established by the Department of Health and the National End of Life Care Programme, and over the next year the group produced a report entitled "End of life care in long term neurological conditions – a framework for implementation". The aim was to encourage health and social care professionals to start to consider end of life issues for this patient group and look at how they could collaborate for the benefit of patients and their families.

This book has arisen from the work in producing the report. The group members have been involved in developing the sections into the chapters. We hope that the book will stimulate services to look at how they can collaborate to improve end of life care, so that the quality of life of patients and their families develop across all areas – elderly care medicine, neurology, rehabilitation medicine, primary care, specialist palliative care, social care and voluntary organisations – and people with neurological disease will receive the co-ordinated and excellent care they require at the end of life.

I would like to thank all the authors involved in this project, those who helped in the production of the original report and the production team at Springer for all their help and enthusiasm in this project.

Rochester, Kent, UK   Dr. David Oliver

Contents

Contributors

Debi Adams, RN, B.A. (Hons) Clinical Nurse Specialist in Palliative Neurology, St. Catherine's Hospice, Scarborough, North Yorkshire, UK

Cynthia Benz, BEd Hons, M.A., Ph.D. Volunteer for the Multiple Sclerosis Society, the National Council for Palliative Care and Dying Matters Coalition, UK

Colin W. Campbell, MBChB, FRCGP, FRCP Medical Director and Palliative Medicine Consultant, St. Catherine's Hospice, Scarborough, North Yorkshire, UK

Debra Chand, B.Sc., M.B.A. The PSP Association, Towcester, Northamptonshire, UK

Barbara J. Chandler, BMedSci, M.B.B.S., M.D., FRCP Raigmore Hospital, Inverness, Scotland, UK

Simon Chapman Director of Policy & Parliamentary Affairs, The National Council for Palliative Care, London, UK

Liz Gwyther, MB ChB, FCFP, M.Sc., Pall Med Hospice Palliative Care Association of South Africa, Pinelands, South Africa

Claire Henry, RGN, PgDip, B.Sc. National End of Life Care Programme, Leicester, Leicestershire, UK

Beverley Hopcutt Therapy Service, Central Manchester University Hospitals NHS Foundation Trust, Manchester, UK

Mark Lee, MBChB, MRCP, M.D. Department of Palliative Care, St Benedict's Hospice & City Hospitals, Sunderland, Tyne and Wear, UK

Susan Mathers, MB ChB, MRCP (UK), FRACP Neurology Unit, Calvary Health Care Bethlehem, Melbourne, Victoria, Australia

David Oliver, B.Sc., FRCP FRCGP Consultant in Palliative Medicine, Wisdome Hospice, Rochester, Kent, UK

Honorary Reader, Centre for Professional Practice, University of Kent, Chatham, Kent, UK

Eleanor Sherwen, RGN, B.Sc. (Hons), Palliative Care, PG Cert ClinEd National End of Life Care Programme, Ongar, Essex, UK

Eli Silber, MBBCh (Wits), FCP (Neuro) SA M.D. (Lond), FRCP Kings College Hospital, London, UK

Jenny Smith, B.Sc. (Hons), MBChB MRCP Specialty Registrar in Palliative Medicine, St Gemma's Hospice, Leeds, Yorkshire, UK

Sue Smith, M.Sc. Motor Neurone Disease Association, Leeds, West Yorkshire, UK

Tes Smith, B.A. (Hons), M.A. Macmillan Cancer Support, Ongar, Essex, UK

Nigel P. Sykes, M.A., FRCP, FRCGP St. Christopher's Hospice, London, UK

Simone Veronese Department of Palliative Care, FARO Foundation, Turin, Italy

Sally Watson, M.A., Ph.D. Director of Executive Education, Lancaster University Management School, Lancaster, Lancashire, UK

Chapter 1
End of Life Care

Tes Smith and Eleanor Sherwen

Abstract The concepts and fields of palliative and end of life care have a long and complex history, and a historical overview both in terms of how death has been viewed in society and some of the changes is helpful in understanding where we are now. This may be linked to the development of the practice of end of life care through the hospice movement and influential events to present day, including the End of Life Care Strategy. The definitions as to end of life and palliative care may be seen as signposts rather than definitive statements. The content of this chapter will in the main be generic as it is acknowledged that the in-depth exploration as to what is end of life care in relation to neurological conditions will contain in the chapters to follow.

Keywords Palliative care • End of life care • Neurological • Overview of care • ELCS

Historical Overview

> Death is both absent and present in contemporary society. There is continuing evidence that we push it away, sometimes shutting it out of sight by the very structures set up in health and social care to deal with dying [1].

The "absent yet present" notion about dying captures many schools of thought around end of life and palliative care. Many books have begun with the historical overview of where palliative medicine, also referred to as palliative care, has been developed from [1–4].

T. Smith, B.A. (Hons), M.A. (✉)
Macmillan Cancer Support,
Ongar, Essex, CM5 0TD, UK
e-mail: tes.smith@me.com; tsmith@macmillan.org.uk

E. Sherwen, RGN, B.Sc. (Hons)
Palliative Care, PG Cert ClinEd,
National End of Life Care Programme,
Ongar, Essex, UK

D. Oliver (ed.), *End of Life Care in Neurological Disease*,
DOI 10.1007/978-0-85729-682-5_1, © Springer-Verlag London 2013

It is the hospice movement that is intrinsically linked to palliative and end of life care by many commentators. A brief exploration regarding the evolution of hospices shows that at the beginning of the nineteenth century hospice care was changing and evolving, having moved from the monasteries providing rest shelter and food in the twelfth to fourteenth centuries to places that cared for the dying from the middle of the seventeenth century onward. Help the Hospices advise caution in comparing the connection between the past and present hospices, in that they reveal hospices in the early times could be said to contain the poor and "downtrodden" and were often places for the spread of diseases and indefinite stays. This is in contrast with the hospices today that tend to focus on short-term care for those close to or at end of their life. Hospices today do vary in the services that offer the local population, many of them offering day therapy, specialist advice and complex symptom management, hospice at home, and psychosocial and bereavement services, to name but a few.

In the UK, the establishment of hospices can be seen in Edinburgh in 1885, followed by several in London: the Hostel of God (now Trinity Hospice) in 1891, Saint Luke Home (latterly St Luke hospital) in 1892, accredited as the site of first medical professional on staff and 1905 saw St Joseph's Hospice Hackney take in its first "patient," a tram driver with incurable lung disease [5]. This time also saw the beginning of the recognition of the need for specialist homes and home care services for those with advanced cancer in the charitable sectors. Hence, The Macmillan Cancer Relief began as the National Society for Cancer Relief in 1911 and the Marie Curie Memorial Foundation in 1948 [5]. Sue Ryder homes began to emerge in the 1970s [6].

These historical markers provide an understanding as to the important connections that have emerged and where and how current thinking has developed. Neuberger, sites death and the wish to have a good death as a concept with its beginnings in ancient times and brings this forward to the Victorian view of a good death being pain free, surrounded by family, prayers and it not being a fearful event [2]. She further suggests that following this the notion and names given to a person approaching death and dying begun to be more obscure and as a result people became less comfortable with death, dying and talking about it. Finally she draws a connection to the brutality and senselessness of war deaths further contributing to the change in attitudes to death and dying, which had turned from a Victorian celebration of life to a culture of not talking about it or telling people that this is in fact what they were "doing" – dying [2]. This obscurity is further borne out by the fact that there are over 200 euphemisms for death in the English language. Dying Matters suggests that the practice of using euphemisms for death is likely to have originated with the belief that to speak the word "death" was to invite death itself. Further it is suggested that this may explain why death is a taboo subject in many English-speaking cultures, and that the use of euphemisms often involves metaphors for the person moving into another state, or another place, which seems to be more acceptable for those dealing with bereavement than using the term "dead" [7].

It has therefore been suggested that by the mid-twentieth century the changes to medicine and health care were having an effect on end of life care. There was increasing emphasis on cure and rehabilitation, while death in hospital as opposed to at home was becoming the norm. Subsequently four significant changes happened:

- A shift in professional literature from anecdote to systemic observation.
- A new way of dying began to emerge, refining ideas about the dying process and exploration as to the extent an individual should know about their condition.
- An active rather than passive approach to the dying was promoted with the encouragement of ways to continue to care for people up to and beyond end of life.
- An increasing awareness of the connections between the physiological and psychological being, thus illuminating the concept of suffering and the need for medical professional need to consider the holistic approach in the treatment of the dying.

When considering a societal approach to death, Kubler-Ross has been attributed with moving the understanding and the culture around death in the late 1960s toward a more "death aware" society, as she recognized that death had become dehumanized and mechanical and called for a rejection of this and a move toward a more proper response to death and dying [8]. Kubler-Ross described a society that had become more interested in the "masses" than the individual and cure and/or keeping alive as opposed to talking the situation through sensitively with the "patient" and enabling discussions around the illness, treatments, and prognosis [9]. It is this discourse that continues to fuel many debates as to who is responsible and when and where should end of life and care planning discussions start. The current thinking on this will be more explored briefly in this chapter and discussed in more detail in subsequent chapters.

It is extensively recognized and documented that Dame Cicely Saunders was instrumental in the emergence of the hospice movement that is currently in place and continues developing today. This work commenced in the 1950s with her initial aspirations to improve the care of those who were dying of malignant disease. Dame Cicely pioneered and developed effective techniques relating to pain control. It was in that field that she recognized and proved the validity and effectiveness of administering analgesia on a regular basis and the positive effects it was having on the lives of those "patients" she was caring for. Dame Cicely Saunders was herself trained in three different professions – nursing, social work, and finally a medical doctor – all in her quest to improve the dying experience for the individual [10]. She opened St Christopher's Hospice in 1967 which is often referred to as the first of the "modern" hospices seeking to combine three key principles: excellent clinical care, education and research, and as a center of excellence in a new field of care. St Christopher's success became the stimulus for hospice development in the UK and abroad and continues to be at the forefront of those same principles today [3].

Therefore, historically attitudes to death and dying changed into one of where death was to be feared rather than celebrated; this correlated with the medical profession pursuing cure for all as opposed to acknowledging when curative interventions were no longer an option. The collision of these changes led to a society and medical profession (among others) that had begun to avoid discussions about death and dying.

In the early 1970s, the first large-scale epidemiological survey led by Professor Ann Cartwright reported on the experiences of people and their families in the last year of life. This was revised in 1987 with a further sample. Several changes were identified; people were:

- Dying alone in increasing numbers
- Older with prolonged and unpleasant symptoms
- In institutional and hospital settings
- Showed a greater awareness of the disease and dying [3]

The latter issue, with regard to greater awareness, is linked to changing practice in the direction of increasing open and honest communication. Holloway notes that there were caveats attached around the basis for that openness in that some people guessed rather than were told they were dying and that people were more likely to have been told about their condition as opposed to being told it would lead to death [1].

The 1980s saw continued growth within this field of palliative care and saw the launch of a scientific journal related to this newly emerging area of medicine and also the recognition of palliative care as a specialist area. In 1985, the Association for Palliative Medicine of Great Britain and Ireland was established. Following further debates, in 1987, palliative medicine was established as a subspecialty of general medicine [3].

The emergence of the speciality oncology in which palliative care is rooted initially showed little interest in the care of the dying according to Clark [3]. 1999 saw the appointment of a cancer tsar – Professor Mike Richards. His role was to reform and improve cancer services building upon the work of the Calman-Hine report and the UK Government's Cancer plan. The Calman-Hine report of 1995 examined cancer services in the United Kingdom and proposed a restructuring of cancer services to achieve a more equitable level of access to high levels of expertise throughout the country. The report further highlighted the need for user involvement by recommending that cancer services should be "patient centered," and the Cancer Plan also recognized this as well as highlighting that cancer services should be a national priority [11]. The outcome was to implement a program of reforms to cancer services which has at its core palliative care services. This work in collaboration with other stakeholders developed the first national strategy for end of life care [3].

This End of Life Care Strategy was published in 2008, with the strap line "promoting high quality care for all adults at the end of life" [12].

The strategy heralded a change to the emphasis placed on end of life care which then became highlighted as one of the eight clinical pathways to be developed by each of the strategic health authorities as part of the "Lord Darzi Next Stage Review." The NHS Confederation noted, "On 3 July 2008 the Department of Health published its vision for primary and community care as part of the NHS Next Stage Review, setting out the future direction for primary and community care in England. NHS Confederation chairman, Bryan Stoten, said: 'This strategy presents opportunities for partners across primary care to work together to improve patient care and this is something that clinicians will be keen to engage with. We know people increasingly want a greater say in their health services and control of their own care'" [13].

The foreword identified that the strategy would provide a framework from which health and social care services could build on [12]. Throughout the message is clear that in order for the actions and recommendations to take shape, health and social care must work together to deliver high-quality care for adults at the end of life. This is a message that remains applicable today in the ever changing landscape of health and social care today, along with the demand for services and the changes in demographics.

A separate review of children's palliative care services was undertaken which resulted in the publication of the first national strategy for children's palliative care – Better care, Better lives [14]. It was suggested that while many issues could be addressed for adults and children in parallel, there were some issues that would have significant differences. These were cited as childhood conditions that cause death before adulthood and the differences as to a child continuing to develop physically, emotionally, and cognitively which affects both health and social care needs. However, the same could also be said of adults, if one subscribes to the concepts suggested by Kubler-Ross that adults do indeed develop and grow through the stages of grief.

The End of Life Care Strategy (adults) highlights in the introduction that around 500,000 people die each year, 99 % of which are over 18 years of age, with most occurring over 65 years of age. Among the conditions these deaths are attributed to are those within the umbrella term of "neurological diseases." This is noted alongside those of heart disease, liver disease, renal disease, diabetes, cancer, stroke, chronic respiratory disease, and dementia [12].

Recent figures have shown that the annual number of deaths is predicted to rise from 503,000 in 2006 to 586,000 in 2030. In 2006, in England and Wales, 290,000 people died in hospital, 95,000 died at home, 47,000 people died in care homes with nursing, 33,000 in other care homes, and 24,000 in hospices [7].

The End of Life Care Strategy identifies and sets out 12 key areas with related actions and recommendations to improve the quality of end of life care in England and Wales:

1. Raising the profile of end of life care
2. Strategic commissioning
3. Identifying people approaching the end of life
4. Care planning
5. Coordination of care
6. Rapid access to care
7. Delivery of high-quality service in all locations
8. Last days of life and care after death
9. Involving and supporting carers
10. Education and training and continuing professional development

11. Measurement and research
12. Funding [12]

The Cicely Saunders Foundation states that although research in the palliative field has grown significantly in the past 15 years, there are important areas yet to be addressed. These areas include barriers to accessing palliative care, supporting services, psychological and spiritual issues, and the care of special groups such as older people and those with different cultural needs. The Foundation concludes that it is the role of palliative care research not just to pose questions but indeed to also offer some answers [10].

Defining End of Life Care Today and Exploring the Remit of Those Who Are Involved in Its Delivery

> We all die; we will all be bereaved. Mostly we don't dwell on this. But death is always a possibility and always has to be dealt with at some point [15].

Singer and Bowman stated in 2002 that the quality of care at the end of life is a global public health issue due to the large number of people involved, and they suggest that if each death affects five other people through care giving and grief, then the number of people affected worldwide by end of life care was in the region of 300 million, equating to 5 % of the world's population [16].

With this in mind, understanding and defining end of life care can be said to be as complex as the concepts they are required to address for an individual. The professionals who work in this field encompass a broad range – those who may be involved in an individual's care will range from highly skilled and trained professionals to those professionals who become involved in this arena of work and to unqualified formal and informal caregivers working in and across a range of settings. The National End of Life Care Programme (NEoLCP) was developed to implement the recommendations of the strategy and has developed a range of practice guidance that seeks to address care provision by different professions within different settings [17]. The strategy identifies the different setting as:

- Acute hospitals
- The community (mainly in a person's home)
- Care homes and sheltered and extra care housing
- Hospices
- Community hospitals
- Ambulance services
- Prisons and secure hospitals
- Hostels for the homeless [12]

The program goes one step further to highlight the importance of recognizing that the physical environments within care settings can have a direct impact on the experiences people have at the end of life and will also impact on the memories of their carers and families. It is also suggested that one issue that is central to care is the importance of providing care settings in which dignity and respect can be facilitated.

As the strategy and policies have developed, further attempts have been made to qualify standards and expectations around the delivery of end of life care. These initially were identified within the Quality Markers for End of Life Care delivery [18]. These were developed alongside the strategy. The National Institute for Health and Clinical Excellence (NICE) is developing these further with 20 standards which encompass all that is necessary to deliver good quality end of life care to an individual and their carers.

These definitions continue to be developed and debated as there continues to be some misunderstanding as to the actual boundaries and depth within both arenas of palliative medicine/care and end of life care. They may be seen as signposts rather than definitive statements and as an attempt to outline the basis of the terms palliative and end of life care. This signposting will also look toward the role professionals play in the delivery of this care and how their role or speciality in this area is held by some professions.

People remain individuals and should be referred to as such rather than as patients. However, people at times do become "patients" in terms of outpatient, inpatient, or GP lists, but throughout their lives, and including their deaths, they remain individual people. It could be suggested that the term "patient" itself can act as a barrier to individualized care and consideration at times, and the term can depersonalize and lead us back to the "masses" mentality suggested by Kubler-Ross. It is a term that is used throughout medical definitions, reports, and strategies, unlike those of social work and social care which alternate often between client, user, and person.

The Royal College of Physicians (RCP) has issued guidance on a number of related topics in conjunction with the management of end of life care in relation to chronic heart failure, lung disease, and renal care and has actively taken part in audits with regard to end of life experiences [19]. They define palliative medicine physicians as:

> Palliative medicine physicians care for patients with life-limiting illnesses, making their lives more comfortable even though their condition is deteriorating. Symptom control is a large part of their work, but they also deal with social and psychological difficulties and get involved in family and carer needs.

> Traditionally, most referrals to palliative care services have been for cancer, but increasingly palliative physicians deal with other illnesses such as end-stage lung, heart and renal disease, and degenerative neurological conditions. The emphasis on rehabilitation and maintenance of function in deteriorating conditions has grown over the years [19].

Further to this, the term palliative care is used widely:

> *Palliative care*: The holistic care of patients with advanced, progressive, incurable illness, focused on the management of a patient's pain and other distressing symptoms and the provision of psychological, social and spiritual support to patients and their family. Palliative care is not dependent on diagnosis or prognosis, and can be provided at any stage of a patient's illness, not only in the last few days of life. The objective is to support patients to live as well as possible until they die and to die with dignity [20].

Initially, it is useful to hold the following as the umbrella understanding as to what it is that the term "end of life" is attempting to capture when used to describe an individual:

> *End of life*: Patients are 'approaching the end of life' when they are likely to die within the next 12 months. This includes those patients whose death is expected within hours or days; those who have advanced, progressive incurable conditions; those with general frailty and co-existing conditions that mean they are expected to die within 12 months; those at risk of dying from a sudden acute crisis in an existing condition; and those with life-threatening acute conditions caused by sudden catastrophic events. The term 'approaching the end of life' can also apply to extremely premature neonates whose prospects for survival are known to be very poor, and patients who are diagnosed as being in a persistent vegetative state (PVS) for whom a decision to withdraw treatment and care may lead to their death [20].

It is also stated that end of life care is that which

> Helps all those with advanced, progressive, incurable illness to live as well as possible until they die. It enables the supportive and palliative care needs of both patient and family to be identified and met throughout the last phase of life and into bereavement. It includes management of pain and other symptoms and provision of psychological, social, spiritual and practical support [12].

For professionals, what does this mean in terms of training and/or professional guidance?

Medical Staff

In 2007, the curriculum for specialist palliative medicine training stated:

> The purpose of this curriculum is to train a specialist in Palliative Medicine.

> Palliative medicine is the branch of medicine involved in the treatment of patients with advanced, progressive, life-threatening disease for whom the focus of care is maximising their quality of life through expert symptom management, psychological, social and spiritual support as part of a multi-professional team. Palliative medicine specialists may work in hospital, in the community and in hospices or other specialist palliative care units [21].

Nurses

For nurses, their role and input within end of life care can occur at many stages in a person's illness. This will include nurses from all sectors, primary, acute, community (including hospitals and care homes), prison, and the private sector. Nurses as with other professionals also practise in many different settings including those outlined above and also in schools and mental health services. In addition to those mentioned above, there are also different strands and specialities of nursing that can be involved at relevant times such as clinical nurse specialists, Macmillan and Marie Curie nurses. To this end, the Royal College of Nurses published in conjunction with the Royal College General Practitioners in England the Charter for End of Life Care in 2011.

The Charter for End of Life Care states that it sets out the best practice standards that all "patients" deserve from their primary health-care team.

The charter further makes seven pledges to "patients" and their families. These pledges are aimed to help people to "live as well as they can, for as long as they can." These pledges include identifying clear communication, helping with choices, preserving dignity, independence, and the term "personal control throughout the course of your illness." Additionally, they outline consulting with others and the writing down and recording of wishes so they are available when required. The word comfortable is also used in the context of care day and night and that specialist care, inclusive of emotional and spiritual needs, is sought for the individual [22].

Social Work

For social work, the beginnings of the profession have been broadly commentated as developing from the almoners. The field of social work and social care is extremely complex. In an attempt to explore this arena, the NEoLCP published Supporting people to live and die well: a framework for social care at the end of life [23]. This framework highlights that social care has a vital role to play in the delivery of end of life care. It also illustrates the role of specialist palliative care social work and that this should be utilized further by mainstream social work and care [23]. Specialist palliative social work has a short history; social workers working in the hospice field came together in the 1980s at St Christopher's and from that meeting and the subsequent identification of the need for an arena of support, the Association of Hospice Social Workers was formed [11]. Beresford et al. offer a full quotation as to how the association describes the field and role of specialist palliative social work. This describes the essence of social work in terms of working with people holistically, from the diverse range of backgrounds and group that represent society today. Additionally, it outlines that social workers are skilled in balancing the needs of those with long-term or life-threatening illnesses alongside those who are bereaved. The core tasks are identified as:

> Specialist palliative care social workers offer a wide range of support to patients and families from practical help with housing and accessing other services through advocacy, individual counselling and group support. This will include bereavement work with adults and children both as individuals and in group settings [11].

Further to this is the identification of what is the guiding principle in social work and in the palliative care field:

> Key to specialist palliative care social work is the desire and ability to see people as whole people and not as a set of problems, to understand the connection of their lives and seek to act on, rather than ignore, the constraints and discrimination they experience in society [11].

Further guidance for allied health professionals who are often part of the wider multidisciplinary team working with those individuals living with and dying from life-limiting conditions is readily found in a variety of sources. The following are examples of these, and this is not intended to be an exhaustive list. No profession or support system has been intentionally overlooked; this is more of an attempt to illustrate many of those who will be involved at some point in the delivery of end of life care. It is also acknowledged that it is the case that some members of professional bodies may not work within the end of life care field per se; however, at some point, they may find themselves working with an individual where end of life care considerations are paramount.

Occupational Therapy

The College of Occupational Therapy has recently worked with NEoLCP to produce guidance for occupational therapists (OTs) working with those at end of life [24]. This publication illustrates the OT role in the delivery of end of life care and serves the dual purpose of giving understanding to OTs in the field and other professionals the contribution OTs can make.

Speech and Language Therapy

The Royal College of Speech and Language Therapists (RCSLT) has provided guidance in relation to their role in end of life care particularly in relation to those individuals living with a diagnosis of head and neck cancers. The 2010 resource manual highlights some key points that begin with acknowledging speech and language therapists (SLTs) are indeed an integral part of a multidisciplinary team working with patients with neurological disease as they have expertise in assessing, diagnosing, and managing disorders of communication, speech, voice, and swallowing. SLTs can develop and support the communication skills of both the individual and others [25], which can be vital at times to ensure communication is retained with the individual where possible.

Physiotherapy

The Chartered Society of Physiotherapy (CSP) has been involved in several publications with regard to the national guidance in terms of end of life care delivery generically. The CSP issued a scope of practice document in 2008; although this does not identify end of life as such, it offers a clear definition as to what physiotherapy is:

> The Curriculum Framework for Physiotherapy (2002) (6) defines physiotherapy as:
> 'A health care profession concerned with human function and movement and maximising potential. It uses physical approaches to promote, maintain and restore physical, psychological and social well-being, taking account of variations in health status. It is

science-based, committed to extending, applying, evaluating and reviewing the evidence that underpins and informs its practice and delivery. The exercise of clinical judgement and informed interpretation is at its core' [26].

It is possible to see that the reference to variations in health status possibly does not adequately identify the role that physiotherapy can have in end of life care and that once again they are a vital part of any multidisciplinary team.

Complementary Therapy

Also, complementary therapy has a role in providing support and comfort to individuals as part of their care plans; this can include massage, acupuncture, reflexology, and hypnotherapy, to name a few. These practitioners have a remit in the delivery of end of life care. They have to date been associated in the main with hospices or private practice although anecdotally we hear of GPs supporting services from the complementary field. Further therapeutic interventions also feature in hospices such as creative art and writing and music therapies [15]. In addition, access to local religious and spiritual leaders is recognized as a need which is appropriate for individuals, carers, and families who express the desire for this support. This support can be vital at both pre- and post-bereavement stages.

Primary Care Team

Within primary care services, there has been increasing awareness of end of life care and the necessity for close involvement in the recognition of the deterioration of the disease process and the approach of death, so that appropriate care can be provided. The Gold Standards Framework in the UK has encouraged general practitioners and the community nursing and other staff to recognize people who may be requiring end of life care. The use of the "surprise questions" – "would you be surprised if this person died in the coming 12 months?" – has been suggested as a way of considering these issues. These principles are increasingly being developed and for neurological conditions certain criteria were suggested for end of life care:

- Progressive deterioration in physical and/or cognitive function despite optimal therapy
- Symptoms which are complex and too difficult to control
- Swallowing problems (dysphagia) leading to recurrent aspiration, pneumonia, sepsis, breathlessness, or respiratory failure
- Speech problems: increasing difficulty in communications and progressive dysphasia
- Specific criteria for MND, PD, and MS [27]

Neurological and Other Specialist Services

Although specialist palliative care and end of life teams may be involved with people with neurological disease as the disease progresses, the principles of end of life care may start much earlier and even from diagnosis [28]. The World Health Organization definition of palliative care suggests:

> An approach that improves the quality of life of patients and their families facing problems associated with life-threatening illness, through the prevention and relief of suffering, early identification and impeccable assessment and treatment of pain and other problems, physical, psychosocial and spiritual. [29]

Thus, for many people with neurological disease, for which there is no curative treatment, palliative care may be appropriate from diagnosis. Moreover, the services and professionals involved at the time of diagnosis can influence the experiences and care later in the disease progression. For instance, a person with MND may hear, soon after diagnosis, of the risks of choking and a distressing death; even though this is not a reality, this may lead to anxiety and distress as the disease progresses [30].

Several teams may be involved in the care of people with neurological disease:

- Neurological services
- Rehabilitation services
- Respiratory or gastrointestinal services – if there are problems with breathing or eating
- Primary care – of the general practitioner and community nurses

They all need to be aware of the issues and prepare the person and their family as deterioration occurs and end of life approaches. Moreover, as cognitive change may occur as the disease progresses – such as in Huntington's diseases or MS – there is a need to discuss difficult issues and advance care planning earlier in the disease [30] (see Chap. 7).

There is increasing awareness within neurological services of the need to consider palliative care and end of life issues. This has been in the USA [31, 32] and the UK [33]. The issues are increasingly included within guidelines [32], and the NICE Guidelines on noninvasive ventilation in MND stressed the importance of discussion about end of life, when commencing noninvasive ventilation [34].

There is a responsibility for all professionals – in health and social care – to be aware of the need to consider end of life issues and work closely together (see Chap. 6).

From all of these, it is possible to see that although the differing professional guidance intention is similar, indeed all professions want the individual to be at the center of all. It is that team approach and joint working between care settings and professionals that at times seems to be lacking. Stark considers the role of the "palliative care consultation team," as she terms it and cites Muir's belief that at the heart of palliative care is the "notion of team" [4]. Stark further suggests that this team should strive to work as an integrated system which can have at its center to ensure the best is achieved for the person and their family. She suggests where and how these teams are involved can depend and vary as to the model that is preferred in a geographical area [4].

The End of Life Care Strategy identifies the need for health and social care to work closely together to deliver the needs of the individual and in passing does identify that a culture change is required to get this delivery right and that this will require efforts from all opinion leaders in all professions and networks [12].

End of Life Care Delivery, What Should It Look Like?

Every life is different from any that has gone before it, and so is every death. The uniqueness of each of us extends even to the way we die [35].

If one does accept and subscribe to the broadly held belief that now as a society we do not talk openly enough about death and dying. And that it is the case that relatively few adults, including older adults, have discussed their own preferences for care with a close relative or friend, making it difficult for others to help ensure their wishes are met. Substantiating this belief, the National Council Palliative Care, through their Dying Matters Coalition, identifies that over 60 % of people have not completed a will, and a recent survey found that although 68 % of people said they were comfortable talking about death, less than a third (29 %) of people have discussed their wishes around dying, and only 4 % have written advance care plans. Around 70 % of people would prefer to die at home, yet of the 500,000 people who die each year in England, around 60 % die in hospitals [36].

Payne cites Corr et al. (2006), who highlighted four areas that people often seek to address during the dying process, a summary of which is provided below:

1. Physical tasks, attending to bodily needs and minimizing physical distress
2. Psychological tasks, achieving autonomy, security, and richness
3. Social tasks, sustaining significant interpersonal attachments
4. Spiritual tasks, identifying, developing, or affirming sources of energy and hope [15]

A barrier to the provision of the above is that it is also often agreed that health and social care staff can often find it difficult to initiate discussions with people about the fact that they are approaching the end of their life or indeed that the condition they are living with is itself life limiting. A question often asked is that, is it that a person's death may be seen as a failure by clinicians and other professionals? Or is it their own fear of death and dying, linked to the prevailing society views that prevent open dialogue? Kubler-Ross observed that in order to sit with someone who is terminally ill without anxiety, we must have considered our own attitude to death and dying [9]. To this view, the strategy can be seen to add that:

How we care for the dying is an indicator of how we care for all sick and vulnerable. It is a measure of society as a whole and it is a litmus test for health and social care services [12].

Kubler-Ross also suggested that "We live in a very particular death-denying society. We isolate both the dying and the old, and it serves a purpose. They are reminders of our own mortality" [37]. She felt that people should not be institutionalized and that we can give more help to people and families with home care nurses and also by giving the family and person "spiritual, emotional, and financial help" to help with the final end of life care at home [37].

It is now widely understood and promoted that a positive way forward for this issue is the need to address with professionals any training needs they may have to assist them overcome their misgivings and enable them to provide what that individual needs and wishes. It is clear that in the absence of open discussions, it is difficult and virtually impossible to elicit people's needs and preferences for care and to plan that care accordingly. The recent prevailing culture of avoidance must now change to ensure that it is the individual and their wishes that are at the forefront or care planning, working in conjunction with the professionals and caregivers to enable the delivery of true person centered end of life care.

In an attempt to address this issue, competences were developed in 2009. This work was completed in partnership by the National End of Life Care Programme, Department of Health, Skills for Care, and Skills for Health. The Common Core Competences and Principles were issued as a guide for health and social care workers working with adults at the end of life. The purpose was to support workforce development, training, and education and the development of new and enhanced roles. The principles and competences attempted to outline and form a common foundation for all of those whose work includes care and support for people approaching or reaching the end of their lives [38, 39].

Additionally, the National End of Life Care Programme has continued to develop and showcase best practice examples; this has been achieved by working with many organizations within health and social care across the many sectors in England, with the continued aim of improving end of life care for adults. One of their main priorities continues to be promoting the need for a joined up approach to care planning and service provision. Moreover, at the heart of all of this practice, development is the need for discussions with the individual to occur in a timely and open way.

One of the issues that continue to be debated is that of when exactly does an individual fall under the umbrella of end of life care? The definition as to when the beginning of end of life care is applicable to an individual is both variable in terms of the individual person and the perspectives of those professionals involved at the time. The strategy itself noted that for some the start would be at time of diagnosis which carries a poor prognosis and cites motor neurone disease as an example of this. It also suggests that a measure could be the use of the surprise question. In that, it may be that some health and social care professionals could find it useful to ask "Would I be surprised if the person in front of me was to die in the next 6 months or year?" If then the answer to this is that they would not be surprised, the next step would be to ask themselves further questions, such as "Is the person likely to be aware of this?" and "Who would be best placed to initiate discussions on the end of life?"

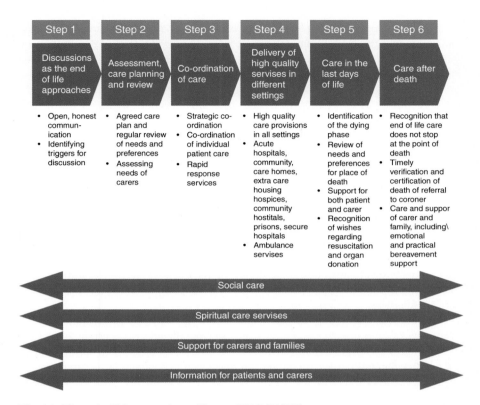

Fig. 1.1 The end of life care pathway (*Source*: NEoLCP [40])

It is further suggested that clinicians in hospital should consider, as they assess a new admission to hospital, about the likelihood of death occurring during that admission [12]. If that is likely then further exploration of that persons wishes should take place alongside the consideration as to whether the admission is really necessary? This would then assist the person in achieving their preferred place of care and ultimately preferred place of death. Therefore, the current prevailing belief is that the earlier these discussions can begin the better, enabling planning and options to be identified and carried out effectively as opposed to crisis managing at the very end of someone's life, when wishes cannot always be achieved.

If we subscribe to the understanding that dying is part of a process and/or pathway, one that a diagnosis leads an individual to, what is it that an individual needs from others to traverse this pathway successfully? In an attempt to address this, the End of Life Care Strategy outlined a care pathway which incorporates a six-step approach (Fig. 1.1). Within each step of the pathway, professionals have distinct roles and duties, and at times, those roles can duplicate and/or merge which does underline the necessity to ensure effective joined up approaches and communication among all those involved in an individual's care.

It must be recognized that each individual will have a different care pathway; no two individual people will have the same needs and preferences. It is understood that many factors will have an impact on an individuals' care needs; these include nature of the condition and its trajectory, living arrangements, social circumstances, preexisting conditions, and/or vulnerabilities, such as mental health issues, experiences of care service to date, experiences of deaths of others, approach to life, and cultural, religious, and spiritual factors.

We are currently in a period of change for many health and social care organizations. This period is seeing many reports being commissioned into how services are being delivered to many different facets of our society and in our communities. The main focus being on the old and vulnerable groups, however, what we know is that we will all die and we only have one chance to get this right for the individual and their carers and families. Those that support and are important to the individual must also feature highly and be considered in all end of life care planning. As Dame Cicely Saunders remarked how we die does remain in people's memories, it also informs people as to how to approach their own demise. This is key to how they may approach any discussions that professionals and caregivers may try to initiate, as if their previous experiences of death have not been positive ones they may wish to avoid discussions.

To conclude, the area of palliative and end of life care has an intriguing and at times checkered history. This, it seems, has been paralleled in the current views held in our society around death and dying. At one level, it is possible to see how much the hospice and palliative care movement has developed and continues to strive for and drive the importance of getting end of life care right. On the other level, the End of Life Care Strategy highlights the work still to be done, yes progress is being made in many areas there is yet more to be done, with specific conditions such as neurological conditions and in the variety of care settings that now provide end of life care.

Dying Matters, Macmillan and other organizations are making strides in raising awareness of these issues. Bringing to the fore the need to have conversation and make plans is vital and must continue. It is recognized that for individuals at times their professional and personal lives may cause a clash in beliefs and therefore practice, it is essential people receive the training and support they need to work with the individuals who are at the end of their lives. This is imperative to ensure we get end of life care right as:

> it is evident that the terminally ill patient has very special needs which can be fulfilled if we take the time to sit and listen and find out what they are [9].

This is also important for family and friends watching their loved ones leave and for the professionals working with them.

It is also important as this will also affect us and have an impact on us when our loved ones die as well as ourselves when we too die.

References

1. Margaret H. Negotiating death, in contemporary health and social care. Bristol: Policy Press; 2007. p. 20–4. 59–60.
2. Julia N. Dying well a guide to enabling a good death. 2nd ed. Oxon: Radcliffe; 2004. p. 1–9.
3. Clark D. From margins to centre: a review of the history of palliative care in cancer. Lancet Oncol. 2007;8:430–8.
4. Altilio T, Otis-Green S. Oxford textbook of palliative social work. Oxford: Oxford University Press; 2011. p. 415.
5. Farleigh Hospice. History of the hospice movement. 2011. www.farliegh.org/about-farleigh-hospice/history-of-farleigh-hospice/. Accessed Aug 2011.
6. National Association of Hospice Fundraisers. History of the hospice movement. 2011. www.nahf.org.uk/what-is-a-hospice/history-of-the-hosice-movement.html. Accessed Aug 2011.
7. Dying Matters. 2011. Source: National Council of Palliative End of Life Care Manifesto 2010. http://www.dyingmatters.org/page/key-facts. Accessed Aug 2011.
8. Haley J. Death and dying opposing viewpoints. Farmington Hills: Greenhaven Press; 2003. p. 10–3.
9. Kubler-Ross E. On death and dying. 240th ed. London: Routledge; 1970. p. 10–34.
10. Cicely Saunders Foundation. About palliative care. 2011, www.cicelysaundersfoundation.org/about-palliative-care. Accessed Aug 2011.
11. Beresford P, Adshead L, Croft S. Palliative care, social work and service users. London: Jessica Kingsley; 2007. p. 26–30.
12. Department of Health. End of life care strategy – promoting high quality care for all adults at the end of life. London: Department of Health; 2008. p. 7–23.
13. NHS confederation. 2011. http://www.nhsconfed.org/OurWork/Policy/NHS-Next-Stage-Review/Pages/The-NHS-Next-Stage-Review.aspx. Accessed Aug 2011.
14. Department of Health. 2008. Better care better lives http://www.dh.gov.uk/en/Publicationsand statistics/Publications/PublicationsPolicyAndGuidance/DH_083106. Accessed Aug 2011.
15. Reith M, Payne M. Social work in end of life and palliative care. 1st ed. Bristol: Policy Press; 2009. p. 29.
16. Singer P, Bowman K. Quality care at end of life should be recognised as a global problem for public health and health systems. BMJ. 2002;324:1291–2.
17. NEoLCP. 2011. www.endoflifecareforadults.nhs.uk/publications. Accessed Aug 2011.
18. Department of Health. End of life care strategy: quality markers and measures for end of life care. 2009. http://www.dh.gov.uk/en/Publicationsandstatistics/Publications/PublicationsPolicy AndGuidance/DH_101681. Accessed Aug 2011.
19. Royal College of Physicians (RCP). Palliative medicine. http://www.rcplondon.ac.uk/specialty/palliative-medicine. Accessed 30 Aug 2011.
20. GMC. Glossary of terms, end of life care. 2011. http://www.gmc-uk.org/guidance/ethical_guidance/end_of_life_glossary_of_terms.asp. Accessed 29 Aug 2011.
21. GMC. Joint Royal Colleges of Physicians Training Board, 2007. 2011. http://www.gmcuk.org/Palliative_medicine_3_Jul_07_v.Curr_0025.pdf_30535465.pdf. Accessed 30 Aug 2011.
22. Royal College of Nurses (RCN). The end of life patient charter. 2011. http://www.rcn.org.uk/__data/assets/pdf_file/0005/386888/EOLC_Charter_FINAL_for_launch_2011_06_01.pdf. Accessed 30 Aug 2011.
23. NEoLCP. Supporting people to live and die well a framework for social care at the end of life 2010. 2011. http://www.endoflifecareforadults.nhs.uk/publications/supporting-people-to-live-and-die-well-a-framework. Accessed Aug 2011.
24. NEoLCP. The route to success – achieving quality for occupational therapy. 2011. http://www.endoflifecareforadults.nhs.uk/publications/rts-ot. Accessed 31 Aug 2011.

25. Royal College of Speech and Language Therapists. Resource manual – head and neck cancers. 2011. http://www.rcslt.org/docs/head_neckfinal. Accessed 31 Aug 2011.
26. The Chartered Society of Physiotherapy (CSP). Scope of practice 2008. 2011. http://www.csp. org.uk/sites/files/csp/secure/PD001%20Scope%20of%20Practice%202008.pdf. Accessed 31 Aug 2011.
27. Thomas K, Sawkins N. The gold standards framework in care homes training programme: good practice guide. Walsall: Gold Standards Framework Programme; 2008.
28. Oliver D. Palliative care. In: Oliver D, Borasio GD, Walsh D, editors. Palliative care in amyotrophic lateral sclerosis- from diagnosis to bereavement. 2nd ed. Oxford: Oxford University Press; 2006.
29. World Health Organization. Palliative care. 2002. www.who.int/cancer/palliative/definition/en/. Accessed Aug 2011.
30. Oliver DJ, Turner MR. Some difficult decisions in ALS/MND. Amyotroph Lateral Scler. 2010;11:339–43.
31. Carver AC, Vickrey BG, et al. End-of-life care: a survey of US neurologists' attitudes, behavior, and knowledge. Neurology. 1999;53(2):284–93.
32. Miller RG, Jackson CE, Kasarskis JD. Practice parameter update: the care of the patient with amyotrophic lateral sclerosis: multidisciplinary care, symptom management, and cognitive/behavioural impairment (an evidence-based review). Neurology. 2009;73:1227–33.
33. EFNS Task Force on diagnosis and management of amyotrophic lateral sclerosis. EFNS guidelines on the management of amyotrophic lateral sclerosis (MALS) – a revised report of an EFNS task force. Eur J Neurol. 2012;19:360–75.
34. National Institute of Clinical Excellence. NICE clinical guideline 105: motor neurone disease; the use of non-invasive ventilation in the management of motor neurone disease. London: NICE; 2010.
35. Nuland S. How we die. 3rd ed. New York: Vintage Books, Random House; 1995.
36. Dying Matters. Source: dying matters NatCen survey, 2009. 2011. http://www.dyingmatters. org/page/key-facts. Accessed Aug 2011.
37. The National Hospice and Palliative Care Organisation (NHPCO). History of hospice care. 2011. www.nhpco.org/i4a/pages/index.cfm?pageid=3285. Accessed Aug 2011.
38. NEoLCP. Core competencies. 2011. http://www.endoflifecareforadults.nhs.uk/publications/corecompetencesguide. Accessed Aug 2011.
39. NICE. Quality standards end of life care – 2011. http://www.nice.org.uk/newsroom/pressreleases/EndOfLifeCareDraftQS.jsp. Accessed Aug 2011.
40. NEoLCP. The route to success in end of life care – achieving quality in prisons and for prisoners. 2011. www.endoflifecareforadults.nhs.uk. Accessed Sept 2011.

Chapter 2
End of Life Care in Neurological Disease

David Oliver and Eli Silber

Abstract Neurological disease may present and progress in many different ways, according to the disease and the individual, and presents a challenge for care throughout the disease progression and particularly at the end of life. These issues include the variability of disease progression, associated cognitive change, complex treatments, and the concerns and problems encountered with inherited diseases. The use of triggers to identify deterioration and the possibility of end of life may be useful in allowing the most appropriate care to be provided, enabling the patient and family to maintain their quality of life.

Keywords Triggers • Palliative care • Recognition of end of life

> **Case Vignette**
>
> Jean was 75 years old and married. She had been diagnosed with Parkinson's disease over 10 years ago but had slowly deteriorated. Her mobility was restricted, and she could only leave the house with help. She was finding eating more difficult, as she could not cook for herself and her swallowing had worsened. She was admitted to hospital on two occasions, following falls at home, but was discharged within 2 days.
>
> On the next occasion, she fell at home and was admitted to hospital. Her condition deteriorated, as she was unable to receive her medication on time. She was restricted to bed but was determined to go home. On discharge, she accepted extra help, but her husband became very tired and found caring for

D. Oliver, B.Sc., FRCP, FRCGP (✉)
Wisdom Hospice,
High Bank, Rochester, Kent, ME1 2NU, UK

Centre for Professional Practice University of Kent, Chatham, Kent, UK
e-mail: drdjoliver@googlemail.com

E. Silber, MBBCh (Wits), FCP (Neuro) SA MD (Lond), FRCP
Kings College Hospital, London, UK
e-mail: eli.silber@nhs.net

D. Oliver (ed.), *End of Life Care in Neurological Disease*,
DOI 10.1007/978-0-85729-682-5_2, © Springer-Verlag London 2013

her more difficult. She was readmitted to hospital and died 2 days later. Her husband and family were shocked, as they had not realized that she was near to the end of her life and had not discussed her wishes with her. They expressed surprise that no health professional had talked of her dying and felt that if they had realized, they would have talked more to her and tried to keep her at home, where she had wished to be.

The care of people with progressive neurological disease provides considerable challenges for clinicians in neurology and palliative care. Neurological diseases offer unique complexities, and while many will share similarities, there are also considerable differences depending on the specific diagnosis. Even in similar conditions, there is considerable variability in the rate of progression, resultant symptoms, and other complications that may ensue. The considerable differences in the rates of progression within the same disease process, and the fact that there are limited biomarkers make prognostication particularly challenging. Thus, there will be great variation as every person is an individual and present with the disease and progress in their own individual particular way.

Neurological diseases have many causes and manifest in very different ways (see Table 2.1).

The main progressive neurological diseases requiring palliative care input are:

- Motor neurone disease
- Multiple sclerosis
- Parkinson's disease and associated diseases:
  - Progressive supranuclear palsy
  - Multiple system atrophy
- Huntington's disease

Neurological services may not always be involved in the diagnosis or ongoing care of people with neurological disease, as acute episodes due to deterioration may be admitted to hospital under the care of other specialities or remain under primary care at home. For instance, stroke is an important acute neurological disease where end of life issues may be of importance, as many patients die acutely in the first episode or are left with severe disability and may deteriorate later, but in the UK, patients are often cared for in stroke units by specialized stroke physicians rather than by neurological services. In most developed countries, brain tumors are also cared for primarily by neurological services, whereas in the UK, the care of this group is primarily within neurosurgical and oncological services. In the majority of developed countries, neurology services are involved in the care of people with dementia, whereas in others, the primary responsibility for directing care is in elderly care or elderly mental care services.

The incidence and prevalence of these diseases varies but overall the numbers of patients requiring care is high. The requirements of care are large and develop over a longer period of time. In England, these common neurological conditions have the

Table 2.1 Diseases of the nervous system that may require palliative care

Central nervous system	
Immune	Multiple sclerosis
	Devic's disease
Infection	HIV
	Creutzfeldt-Jakob disease
	Subacute sclerosing panencephalitis
Degenerative	Motor neurone disease
	Parkinson's disease
	Progressive supranuclear palsy
	Multiple system atrophy
	Alzheimer's disease and other dementias including frontotemporal (Pick's)
	Cerebellar degenerations
Inherited	Huntington's disease
	Inherited cerebellar ataxias
	(Autosomal dominant – SCAs and recessive Friedreich's ataxia)
Vascular	Stroke (infarction and hemorrhage)
	Subarachnoid hemorrhage
Severe acute acquired injury	Hypoxia
	Traumatic – brain and spinal injury
Neoplastic	Primary brain tumors
	Metastatic disease
	Paraneoplastic syndromes (cerebellar, limbic encephalitis)
Peripheral nervous system	
Anterior horn cell disease	Postpolio syndrome
Peripheral nerve disease	Inherited – Charcot-Marie-Tooth disease
	Amyloid
	Inflammatory – Guillain-Barre/CIDP
	Paraneoplastic neuropathies
	Neuropathies associated with chronic conditions
Neuromuscular junction disease	Lambert-Eaton syndrome
	Myasthenia gravis
Muscle disease	Inherited dystrophies (e.g., Duchenne muscular dystrophy)
	Inherited myopathies

following prevalence and total numbers of patients and account for these numbers of deaths:

	Prevalence	Estimated numbers[a]	Annual deaths[b]
Parkinson's disease	110–180/100,000	120,000	7,700
Multiple sclerosis	110–140/100,000	100,000	1,500
Motor neurone disease	6/100,000	5,000	1,500
Huntington's disease	6–10/100,000	5,000	240
Multiple system atrophy	5/100,000	4,500	200
Progressive supranuclear palsy	6/100,000	5,000	310

[a]Assuming England of population 50 million
[b]The condition is mentioned on the ONS return from the death certificates during the period 2002–2010 [1]

Clinical Approach to Palliative Care for Neurological Patients

The specific needs of neurological patients will vary according to diagnosis, stage of progression, and individual characteristics. However, there are some needs and concerns that will be common to many patients and their families, particularly at the end of life. There will be similarities across disease groups in the issues faced, and will require a palliative care approach. The World Health Organization defines palliative care as:

> An approach that improves the quality of life of patients and their families facing problems associated with life-threatening illness, through the prevention and relief of suffering, early identification and impeccable assessment and treatment of pain and other problems, physical, psychosocial and spiritual [2]

Moreover, The UK National End of Life Care Strategy [3] suggests a pathway for end of life care comprising six steps – see Chap. 2 page x. Neurological diseases are included in the chronic illnesses considered within the strategy [3]. The strategy also stresses that people at the end of life should have access to:

- The opportunity to discuss needs and preferences and record them in a care plan
- Coordinated care and support
- Rapid specialist advice and assessment
- High-quality care and support during the last days of life
- Services which treat people with dignity and respect before and after death
- Appropriate advice and support for carers at every stage

These ideals are still being developed but challenge all services involved in the care of patients with progressive disease.

Neurological diseases have considerable differences in their care and support compared to other advancing disease – in particular cancer, which is often considered the basis of the palliative care approach. The main differences are:

1. The broad spectrum of neurological conditions leading to the challenges of diagnosis – which may be delayed and lead to advanced disease at the time of diagnosis and prognosis.
2. Variable rate of progression.
3. Mixture of cognitive and physical disability.
4. The overlap between physical, communication, cognitive, and mental health issues resulting in considerable management challenges.
5. Complex diseases, in some the diagnosis may be difficult and delayed because of an inability to biopsy and no clear biomarkers.
6. Some neurological conditions are inherited affecting the responses and concerns of families.
7. Recognition of end of life care. Many patients can live with severe disability for some time, and it may be difficult to recognize when palliative care is required.

There are a large number of neurological disorders; in most, palliative care is unnecessary and inappropriate, and in others, it is important.

Variability in Progression

Neurological conditions are widely variable, and thus planning end of life care can prove challenging.

The changes may be:

- Acute onset, death, or variable recovery – as in stroke or trauma
- Rapid decline over months/a few years – such as MND
- Prolonged deterioration over several years – Huntington's disease, Parkinson's disease, PSP, and MSA
- Fluctuating condition with variable needs – such as MS

In some patients, the requirement for palliative care is both inevitable and fairly rapid, and in others, only a minority will require specialist palliative care on a longer term basis but may require care at the end of life. The progressive nature and the limited prognosis of motor neurone disease will often mean that it is appropriate to involve and plan palliative care from the time of diagnosis [4]. However, for some conditions, although they are progressive, the rate of progression may vary from months to decades. For instance, for the primary degenerative conditions such as Parkinson's disease or multiple sclerosis, the prognosis is generally good with only a limited average effect on longevity, but palliative care input may be required for those with a particularly severe disease course and when there is a final deterioration at the very end of life. For some diseases, the requirements are almost inevitable, and in others, only the most severely affected patients may require palliative care.

It is helpful to make a distinction between palliative care skills that should be part of the repertoire of all GPs, physicians, and neurologists, particularly those with an interest in the management of patients with chronic conditions, and specialist palliative care, which may be required for more complex and difficult situations – complex symptom management issues or psychosocial issues. It is also recognized that in the management of people with advanced neurological conditions, the neurologist may have specific and essential knowledge and skills, such as in the management of spasticity, adjustment of Parkinson's medication, and treatment of autonomic dysfunction, making their input valuable even when the patients are in the later stages of disease progression. End of life for neurological patients therefore almost inevitably requires the collaboration of those with expertise in palliative care working with those with neurological expertise (neurologists, elderly care physicians, rehabilitation consultants, psychiatrists, and nurse specialists) if the quality of life for people with neurological conditions is to be maximized.

New attitudes to patient autonomy and new ways of team working may be needed to ensure that patients' wishes are central to care plans and that each member of the team is clear about their roles and responsibilities. In comparison to palliative care for

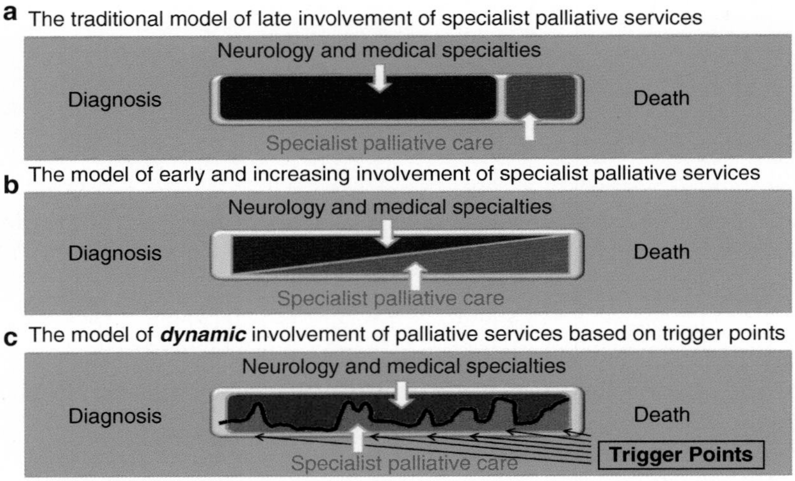

Fig. 2.1 Palliative care services and involvement in neurological disease (Taken from Bede et al. [6])

terminal cancer patients, as the person's needs vary over time, there may be a role for episodic involvement of palliative care services during the progression of the disease. This may occur at times of particular distressing symptoms, when patients face change or when psychosocial issues arise. Such times include diagnosis, the commencement of an intervention such as gastrostomy or ventilator support, or at the very end of life. This may be a challenge for all concerned, to ensure that coordinated care is maintained with good communication among the various professionals involved.

This change in involvement and the need for care to vary over time can be challenging for all the caring teams. Conventionally palliative care services have become involved in the person's care and remained an integral part of the care pathway until death (Fig. 2.1). In the past, this may have been after a clear decision from "curative" to "palliative" care, particularly for a cancer patient – model 1. However, this has not been a sustainable system as many patients receive palliative chemotherapy even during the later stages of life, aiming at improving quality of life rather than extending life. This same pattern would apply for other advancing illnesses, and a pathway of integrated care is often seen – with reducing curative/active treatment as palliative care increases – model 2 [5].

Neurological diseases, with varying prognosis and varying needs, may require a new model of care – model 3 – in which palliative care/end of life care services have an episodic involvement with less contact between these phases of care [5, 6]. For instance a person with MND may need greater involvement at the time of diagnosis – coping with the shock of the diagnosis; and thereafter at points of transition, such as at the time of consideration of wheelchair or other aid for living; at the time of consideration of gastrostomy; when ventilatory support, by noninvasive ventilation or invasive ventilation with a tracheostomy, is being considered; at the end of life over the final weeks/days of life.

These models are shown in Fig. 2.1. Model 3, with episodic involvement, may be more appropriate for neurological disease as the needs vary over time. However, there is also increasing awareness that the same model of care may be appropriate for people with advancing cancer, heart disease, or respiratory disease as there is increasing active/disease modifying care and only specific phases, which may be seen as triggers, for palliative care involvement.

The variability can be very difficult for all involved in the care of a person with neurological disease. For some people, there may be a long disease progression with great variability in the functional and mental ability of the person – such as with MS – and the sudden deterioration, perhaps with an infection that does not on this occasion respond to treatment, may be a shock to all concerned.

The experience of palliative care in dealing with difficult discussions about the diagnosis or management and treatment options and advance planning means that they have a potentially valuable role from both relatively early in the process and then at later as the disease progresses.

Specific Issues, Autonomy, and Complexity

Mixture of Cognitive and Physical Disability

Many people with neurological disease face altered autonomy which may be due to – changes in mood, cognitive abilities, communication, due to dysphasia or dysarthria, or more complex neuropsychiatric problems, such as:

- Dementia in MS
- Frontal lobe dysfunction or frontotemporal dementia (FTD) in MND
- Dementia in Parkinson's disease (Lewy body dementia)
- Severe cognitive change in Huntington's disease
- Hallucinations and psychiatric changes in PSP or Parkinson's disease
- Impulsivity or loss of judgment in dementia or PD
- Behavioral changes – in dementia, PSP, MS, MSA, and PD and FTD in MND

There is the potential of these changes to affect how end of life care is planned, and they can cause distress to patients, families, and professional carers, as the person may be very different to their previous personality or behaviour.

It may be necessary for people to discuss their wishes earlier in the disease progression, while they have the capacity to do so. Delaying until later in the disease may not be feasible, as they may then be unable to express their views clearly – due to communication or cognitive issues. However, this earlier discussion may be difficult for all concerned – patient, family, and professionals – help may be needed to allow the discussion and expression of the views to be made – and advance care planning arranged – see Chap. 7.

Complex Treatments

Some patients may receive complex interventions. These may include medication to treat the disease such as Parkinson's disease therapy, cytotoxics, and monoclonal antibodies in MS or symptomatic therapies. They often also include more invasive therapies treatments such as deep brain stimulation in Parkinson's disease or ventilator support in MND, either as noninvasive ventilation or more rarely invasive ventilation with a tracheostomy. These interventions often lead to complex ethical issues [7]. There may be disease progression and treatment may no longer be appropriate or acceptable to the person, and withdrawal of treatment may be discussed. The wider multidisciplinary team will face challenges in helping patients and their families in these difficult decisions and in supporting each other during these discussions. There is a challenge of working with/integrating the various teams and dealing with patients' expectations to decide when these complex therapies no longer extend life or improve quality of life, and when care needs to be predominantly palliative, i.e., "knowing when to stop."

Disease-Specific Problems

Parkinson's Disease (PD) and Other Parkinsonian Syndromes

PD is a progressive condition, but with modern dopamine replacement therapy, symptoms can be controlled for several years, and life expectancy for people with PD can approach normal. However, most patients will suffer a progressive decline prior to end of life due to motor fluctuations, excessive dyskinesias, nonmotor complications including neuropsychiatric problems, both mood, hallucinations, and cognition, as well as autonomic dysfunction.

More complex treatments are possible and may be considered:

- Different means of receiving drug – apomorphine infusion/duodenal dopamine.
- Deep brain stimulation.
- Stem cell transplantation – this is still an area of research and its value is undetermined.

While there are a number of treatment modalities to consider in this situation, palliative care should be involved as the disease progresses and conventional therapies fail to help with symptom management. Patients should be encouraged to undertake advance care planning but they, their carers, and clinicians need to be aware that patients can deteriorate dramatically and may appear close to death due to treatment problems, and/or intercurrent infections, only to recover swiftly with appropriate treatment and resume their previous way of life. A Parkinson's disease specialist should be able to advise on optimal and appropriate treatment and what can be achieved in these circumstances.

Initially, it may be difficult to distinguish Parkinson's disease from other Parkinsonian syndromes, multiple system atrophy, and progressive supranuclear palsy. In MSA, there is a combination of Parkinsonism with pyramidal, cerebellar, and autonomic dysfunction. Similarly, PSP combines Parkinsonism with other features including limitation of eye movements, gait instability, cognitive loss, and autonomic failure resulting often in tendency to fall. The prognosis of these conditions is considerably worse (approximately 5 years from diagnosis), and almost all patients develop considerable disability requiring complex care, including palliative care.

Multiple Sclerosis (MS)

In the majority of people with MS (80 %), the disease initially has a relapsing course with attacks affecting different parts of the central nervous system, particularly the optic nerves, brain, and spinal cord. Initially, there is complete or partial recovery between attacks, but after 10 years or so, approximately half will eventually decline, a condition termed secondary progression. About 20 % will have primary progression from the onset. In the relapsing phase of the disease, disease-modifying therapies may be used to reduce relapses and therefore the risk of permanent disability. These therapies are thought to be ineffective in the progressive phases of the disease, and a proportion of patients will develop profound disability.

In most patients, the effects on longevity are limited; in some, the disease can result in severe relapses, rapid progression, and early disability. Patients can develop complex problems with pain; mobility problems and spasticity; fatigue; skin, bowel, and bladder care difficulties; communication and swallowing problems; and psychiatric and cognitive complications. Death related to MS is usually due to respiratory complications from dependency or other complications of immobility. In contrast to cancer, many patients will live for years with severe disability, and the stage when palliative care involvement may be required may well be protracted and the duration difficult to predict.

Motor Neurone Disease (MND)

While for many people with MND, the course is predictable and palliative care can be planned in a similar way to the paradigm for cancer patients, other patients can die suddenly from respiratory collapse without specific warning, and a small group (about 10 %) have a slowly progressive form of MND which can last 10–20 years.

Increasingly new treatments are used in the care of people with MND, in particular:

- Riluzole – a medication that has been shown to reduce the rate of decline of the disease progression but does not alter the disease itself. Often patients wish to

continue with the medication even after there has been profound progression and
its use may no longer be appropriate
- A gastrostomy tube for feeding when there is severe dysphagia – either a percutaneous endoscopic gastrostomy (PEG) or a percutaneous radiological gastrostomy (PRG) may be inserted. This will allow nutrition and medication to be
  continued when swallowing is difficult and improves quality of life. However, as
  the patient approaches end of life, the use of nutrition and hydration through the
  gastrostomy may become less appropriate. Careful discussion about the reduction or withdrawal of fluids may be necessary.
- Noninvasive ventilation (NIV) is increasingly used to relieve the symptoms of
  respiratory muscle weakness, leading to respiratory failure. However, the disease
  will still progress, with increasing disability and problems, and the patient may
  become more dependent, and on occasions totally dependent on ventilatory support. Discussion about withdrawal of the ventilator may be necessary.
- On occasions, patients with MND may present acutely with respiratory failure and
  an uncertain diagnosis, and a tracheostomy with invasive ventilation is commenced.
  The patient can be maintained for long periods of time, with increasing disease
  progression and disability and with the risk of becoming totally locked in – with no
  communication. Discussion of withdrawal of ventilation may be necessary, and
  forward advance care planning will allow the person control of their care, even if
  they have lost capacity to communicate – see Chap. 7.

Other Conditions

Other conditions including those of the peripheral nervous system can each pose
their specific challenges, e.g., muscular dystrophy and progressive neuropathies. In
many, the onset is at a younger age, and cognition is preserved, making these a particularly challenging and rewarding group of patients to care for. The nervous system is affected by malignancies in three ways. This includes primary brain tumors,
metastatic tumors to the brain, and paraneoplastic conditions where the nervous system is affected by the body's immune response to an underlying malignancy. Again
consideration needs to be given to the specialist management, involvement of a
multidisciplinary team, and close liaison with palliative care when required.

Some of the clinical issues for each disease group are shown in Table 2.2.

The pathway shown below (Fig. 2.2) suggests that all patients should be regularly assessed for the various triggers that may suggest that there is a significant
deterioration in their condition and that end of life issues need to be considered.
From the initial diagnosis of a life-limiting condition, it is important that the changes
in disease progression are recognized in all care settings as triggers for the introduction and subsequent stepping up and stepping down of palliative care input, based
on holistic assessment which includes the needs of careers, joined-up planning,
good communication, and regular review.

Table 2.2 Common issues/triggers for progressive neurological diseases

Condition	Specific issues
Multiple sclerosis	Depression
	Spasms
	Cognitive change
	Dysphagia with reduced hydration and nutrition
	Skin fragility and increased risk of pressure sores
	Mobility problems
Parkinson's disease	Rigidity
	Pain
	Agitation/confusion from sepsis
	Neuropsychiatric decline
Motor neurone disease	Respiratory failure or increased breathlessness
	Reduced mobility
	Dysphagia
Multiple system atrophy	Aspiration pneumonia
	Depression
	Hallucinations/anxiety/psychosis from neuropsychiatric decline
Progressive supranuclear palsy	Depression
	Cognitive and behavioral change
	Visual impairment
	Reduced mobility
	Spasms
	Dysphagia

Recognition of End-of-Life Care

Identifying when someone with advanced neurological condition may be approaching the end of life care phase of their illness is important because it enables the appropriate care to be planned. It is important in those people who have lived with chronic disability to distinguish this from deterioration, due to an intercurrent illness.

However, there are often occasions when the triggers which could suggest that end of life should be considered are not recognized or even ignored. These include:

- The patient may not wish to discuss these issues or may have cognitive changes (which may or may not be recognized) that make the discussion more difficult.
- The family and close carers may not wish to face the reality of the deterioration and affect the opportunities to discuss these issues.
- The health and social care professionals may not be experienced enough or willing to recognize the triggers or changes they see – due to their close involvement with the patients and family, or their own personal views.
- The health and social care professionals may be reluctant to discuss these issues.
- The transition to end of life care may be so gradual and insidious that it is not recognized by the person or their carers.

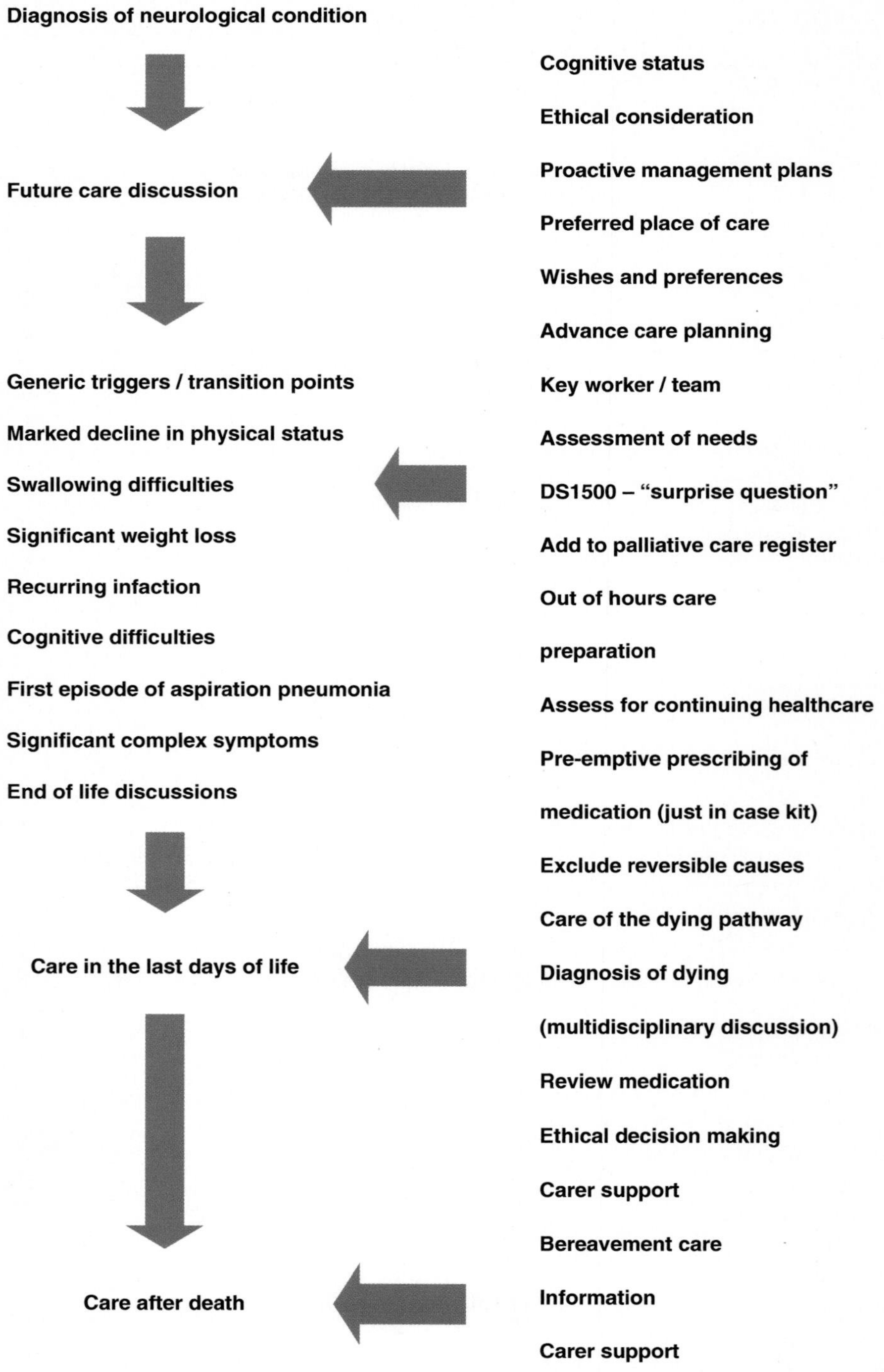

Diagnosis of neurological condition

Cognitive status

Ethical consideration

Future care discussion   Proactive management plans

Preferred place of care

Wishes and preferences

Advance care planning

Generic triggers / transition points   Key worker / team

Marked decline in physical status   Assessment of needs

Swallowing difficulties   DS1500 – "surprise question"

Significant weight loss   Add to palliative care register

Recurring infaction   Out of hours care

Cognitive difficulties   preparation

First episode of aspiration pneumonia   Assess for continuing healthcare

Significant complex symptoms   Pre-emptive prescribing of

End of life discussions   medication (just in case kit)

Exclude reversible causes

Care of the dying pathway

Care in the last days of life   Diagnosis of dying

(multidisciplinary discussion)

Review medication

Ethical decision making

Carer support

Bereavement care

Care after death   Information

Carer support

Fig. 2.2 End-of-life care pathway for neurological disease (Adapted from National End of Life Care Programme [9])

There is the need for all involved to consider the issues, and there may need to be further developments within society to facilitate the openness to facing deterioration and death. *Dying Matters* [8] aims to encourage these discussions more widely in society and hopefully will open up these areas for wider discussion for all involved. This will also include greater awareness of the need to consider and discuss end of life issues by all the professionals involved. Although some team members may feel able to discuss these issues, others may not, and there may be a need to encourage greater discussion and openness with all the health and social care professionals involved.

The attitudes of professionals may vary greatly – due to education, personal experience, cultural or religious attitudes and experience. Greater awareness and discussion may require some professionals to alter their own attitudes and be aware of the particular needs and wishes of their patients. Education and greater discussion within all teams may help encourage this openness and awareness of patient and family needs. Integration of palliative care into teams will help considerably.

The End of Life Care Pathway [3] – see Chap. 1 page x – suggests consideration of end of life care throughout the disease progression, and the UK National End of Life Care Programme "Improving end of life care in long term neurological conditions – a framework for implementation" suggests certain triggers when end of life issues should be considered (Fig. 2.2). There are generic triggers for all neurological diseases:

- Swallowing problems
- Recurrent infection – particularly respiratory infection that may be associated with aspiration
- Marked decline in physical status – generalized weakness and reduced mobility and activity
- First episode of aspiration pneumonia
- Cognitive difficulties – confusion or more subtle cognitive change
- Weight loss
- Significant complex symptoms:

  Pain
  Spasticity
  Nausea
  Psychosocial or spiritual issues

The recognition of these issues may alert professionals that there has been significant deterioration, necessitating a change in emphasis in management perhaps from a more investigative and active management approach to a palliative approach. Some symptoms may be reversible in some circumstances – such as with an intercurrent infection, period of depression, or inadequate medication – and in all cases, it is important to identify and treat any reversible problems.

There may be specific triggers for a particular disease but it is essential to consider every patient individually, as there will be great variation in the disease progression and needs between patients, even with the same disease. The specific triggers for the main progressive diseases are shown in Table 2.2 [9].

Recognition and further discussion among the team – patient (if possible), family and close carers, and the wider multidisciplinary team – may then allow the management plan to consider the possibility that this person may be deteriorating and coming to the end of life. In this way, the care provided can be more appropriate and advance care planning and preparation for the end of life may start – as described in later chapters.

Conclusion

The care of people with neurological disease, particularly at the end of life, is complex and involves many different disciplines and teams. There is the need to recognize the needs of patients and their families throughout the disease progression and identify and recognize the triggers that may indicate that there is significant deterioration requiring a palliative approach to improve the quality of life as the end of life comes nearer.

References

1. National End of Life Care programme. NEoLC intelligence network bulletin: deaths from neurodegenerative diseases in England 2002–2008. 2010. Access at www.endoflifecare-intelligence.org.uk. Accessed 14.4.12.
2. World Health Organization. Palliative care. 2002. www.who.int/cancer/palliative/definition/en/. Accessed 14.4.12.
3. National End of Life Care Strategy for England. London, UK: Department of Health. 2008. www.dh.gov.uk/en/Publicationsandstatistics/Publications/PublicationsPolicyAndGuidance/DH_086277. Accessed 17.4.12.
4. Oliver D. Palliative care. In: Oliver D, Borasio GD, Walsh D, editors. Palliative care in amyotrophic lateral sclerosis – from diagnosis to bereavement. 2nd ed. Oxford: Oxford University Press; 2006.
5. Maddocks I, Brew B, Waddy H, Williams I. Palliative neurology. Cambridge: Cambridge University Press; 2006.
6. Bede P, Hardiman O, O'Brannagain D. An integrated framework of early intervention palliative care in motor neurone disease as a model to progressive neurodegenerative diseases. Poster at European ALS Congress, Turin. 2009.
7. Oliver DJ, Turner MR. Some difficult decisions in ALS/MND. ALS. 2010;11:339–43.
8. Dying Matters. National council for palliative care. www.dyingmatters.org. Accessed 28.4.12.
9. National End of Life Care Programme. End of life care in long term neurological conditions – a framework for implementation. 2010. http://www.endoflifecareforadults.nhs.uk/assets/downloads/neurology_report___final___20101108_1.pdf. Accessed 17.4.12.

Chapter 3
Communication

Jenny Smith, Debi Adams, and Colin W. Campbell

Abstract Communication between the patient and professional as equals is essential in supporting people with progressive neurological conditions. The outcome of good communication in end of life care is to return a sense of control to the person. It can increase the person's understanding of what may happen as their disease progresses and empower them to make important choices for their future care. Supporting effective communication in end of life care for people with neurological disease is challenging, but there are common themes in doing this well. Involvement of speech and language therapy services is important for assessment of speech problems and planning communication support.

   This chapter describes the physical and cognitive problems which can compound communication difficulties in neurological diseases. Strategies to support effective communication in these situations are offered, particularly for giving the initial diagnosis of the disease and understanding and assessing signs of distress in individuals with cognitive impairment, and the anticipation and early recognition of communication problems are identified as triggers for future care planning. Sensitively exploring the person's end of life wishes is one area in which good communication is central to returning control. These important discussions can enable the individual to determine where and how they would like to be treated as their disease progresses. The essence of good communication in neurological disease is to firstly focus on the person, not the disease, and to promote individual choice and control.

Keywords Communication • Cognition • Speech • Diagnosis • Questions • Capacity

J. Smith, B.Sc., (Hons), MBChB MRCP(✉)
Specialty Registrar in Palliative Medicine, St. Gemma's Hospice,
329 Harrogate Road, Moortown, Leeds, Yorkshire, LS17 6QD, UK
e-mail: smithjen69@hotmail.com

D. Adams, RN, BA (Hons)
Clinical Nurse Specialist in Palliative Neurology, St. Catherine's Hospice,
Throxenby Lane, Scarborough, North Yorkshire, UK

C.W. Campbell, MBChB, FRCGP, FRCP
Medical Director and Palliative Medicine Consultant, St. Catherine's Hospice,
Throxenby Lane, Scarborough, North Yorkshire, UK

D. Oliver (ed.), *End of Life Care in Neurological Disease*,
DOI 10.1007/978-0-85729-682-5_3, © Springer-Verlag London 2013

Harry's Story

Harry was in the advanced stages of multiple system atrophy. His speech was incomprehensible to most people. Some words could be guessed correctly with much repeating. Despite his great difficulty speaking, Harry seemed able to communicate so much with his eyes and wide smile. He could let you know that you understood him or even just that he was pleased to be with you and hear some gossip. His wife, Ann, was able to understand more than most what he was saying, but now, even she struggled to understand him. Earlier in his disease, Harry had been quick at using his communication boards, but increased weakness meant that even these simple aids were proving difficult to use. He was becoming weaker quickly and was now struggling to eat anything, managing only a couple of spoonfuls of his supplement puddings at a time, and drinking very little.

One year before, Harry had a severe chest infection due to aspiration and was admitted to hospital. He was more able to speak in those days, and when he returned home, he let his GP know that he did not want to be taken into hospital again. He said he felt "lost" in hospital and he felt he did not want to be "kept alive." Harry met with a specialist palliative care nurse and consultant, and his future wishes were explored. Harry knew his swallowing reflex was failing and he was losing weight. He stated very clearly that he did not want to have a feeding tube and did not ever want to go to hospital again. While he knew his wife would need help, he wanted to stay at home.

Ann was terribly worried. She knew Harry was dying, but she was concerned that he was suffering in hunger, in thirst, and in pain. Ann phoned the specialist nurse who visited that day. Harry was in bed and unable to move at all. Ann was distressed. "He hasn't eaten or drunk anything today…I can't bear not to be able to help him." Ann had been sitting for hours with Harry, trying to get him to take some food. She was exhausted. "Anything I put in his mouth just falls out." Ann explained that Harry had been managing to blink once for "yes" and twice for "no" but that today even this seemed too much effort for him. The nurse said she would like to try and talk with Harry to find out how he was feeling and what he wanted. Harry's fingers were fixed into fists, and the nurse puts two of her fingers into the center of his right fist.

Nurse: "Harry, I would like to try and understand if there is anything you want to tell us. I wonder if you can squeeze my fingers?"

Harry: Slowly, Harry squeezed the nurse's fingers.

Nurse: "Can you squeeze my fingers once for 'yes'?"

Harry: one squeeze

Nurse: "Now can you try and squeeze twice that can be for 'no'?"

Harry: two squeezes

Nurse: "Harry, I understand that you are weaker and that eating and drinking are very difficult. It seems that your condition has progressed considerably, and I'm sorry that you may not recover. Do you understand what I am saying? Can you squeeze my fingers once for 'yes' and twice for 'no' if you understand?"

Harry: one squeeze

Nurse: "I know you have said before that if you became unwell, you would not want to go to hospital. You also said that you would not want treatment to prolong your life anyway. Can you let me know if this is still how you feel? Can you squeeze my hand once for 'yes' and twice for 'no'?"

Harry: one squeeze

Nurse: "I understand you feel some distress. Are you hungry?"

Harry: two squeezes

Nurse: "Are you feeling thirsty?"

Harry: one squeeze

Nurse: "There are some things we can do to help relieve your thirst, maybe some moistened sponges around your mouth and a saliva replacement mouth spray. Would you like to try these?"

Harry: one squeeze

Ann becomes concerned that he should receive fluids by tube feeding as he is getting dehydrated. The nurse explains that the need for fluid may decrease as the person deteriorates and the aim would be to provide comfort by using sprays of water or sponges to keep his mouth moist. Harry goes on to communicate that the main distress he feels is from pain caused by significant stiffness throughout his body. He agrees to have midazolam in a syringe driver to relieve the pain of stiffness. Harry lets Ann know that he is not worried or frightened about anything and she shouldn't worry about him.

Two days later, Harry died peacefully in his own bed. Ann said, "He just seemed to gradually drift off into a deeper and deeper sleep, and in the end, he just didn't wake up. I feel so lost without him, but I'm glad for his sake, it is all over."

Introduction

> I stiffened my body and put my left foot out again, for the third time. I drew one side of the letter. I drew half the other side…I set my teeth so hard that I nearly pierced my lip. But – I drew it – the letter "A"…shaky, with awkward wobbly sides and a very uneven centre line… I had done it! I had started – the thing that was to give my mind its chance of expressing itself…my road to a new world, my key to mental freedom [1].

The above quote from the poet and author Christy Brown, using his toes to write, illustrates how even a simple technique can be a powerful tool in communication and an opportunity for personal expression. Despite profound changes in the quality of speech, there are a range of methods and strategies that can enable patients to communicate.

When talking about end of life care with people who have neurological conditions, the focus must firstly be on the person rather than the disease itself. It is a priority to gain understanding of the individual's personality, worries, and wishes. "In the absence of a curative treatment, it is the individual rather than the disease that must be cared for." [2]

There are significant communication challenges as a result of the physical and cognitive impairments of neurological conditions. However, a wide range of approaches, techniques, and strategies can assist in supporting individual choice, gaining understanding, and building relationships.

Communication Problems in Neurological Disease

Speech Problems

Speech problems can lead to ineffectual communication, resulting in feelings of isolation, depression, and loss of control.

Communication is a two-way process, and effective communication is important as it allows us to learn about an individual and allows them to convey their thoughts and wishes in order to maintain a positive quality of life and psychosocial well-being [3]. Communication conveys emotion and allows us to express opinions and exert control over our environment. Speech is a reflection of personality in terms of who an individual is, where they originate from, what they like, and what is important to them. When someone's speech changes, it not only affects how they communicate but also how they feel as a person and how others react to them.

> I rely on this Lightwriter (artificial means of communicating verbally) now, as I can no longer speak. I used to have a strong, loud Geordie accent which everyone recognised as me before I even entered the room. Now I sound like a robot with no emotion. I feel that people treat me differently now and I hate it when they try to guess what I am typing. (63-year-old man with MND)

The physiology of speech production requires precise coordination between breathing, vocal cords, and muscles of the tongue, lips, and mouth. If there is disturbance of the neurological input to any of these muscles, this may result in difficult or incomprehensible speech.

Many of the neurological disorders have the potential to affect speech and communication. This may be one of the first symptoms noticed before help is sought and a diagnosis is eventually made, often some months later. Speech problems are often subtle at first and may become progressively worse as the condition deteriorates and are often overshadowed by the more predominant motor symptoms. There can be variation in severity of impairment over a few hours if the person is tired. Gradual changes to the speech process may occur over months as the disease changes or if there is concurrent illness.

There is a certain stigma attached to speech impairment, and the development of speech problems can be embarrassing for the individual. As conversation becomes more difficult, they may start to withdraw from social situations to avoid any embarrassment and upset. Taking the lead in conversations or following fast-changing topics can be very problematic for those with speech problems. It can certainly make more in-depth and complex discussions difficult unless thought has been given to support measures for the patient. This support can take the form of simply allowing more time or speech aids and will be discussed further in this chapter.

Speech problems can be anticipated in some neurological disorders. There should therefore be discussions about planning with the patient and carer, empowering them to remain at the center of all discussions. Speech problems can be progressive, but in many of the neurological disorders, the speed of deterioration is sufficiently slow to allow time to recognize the problem and devise strategies to cope. If wishes and concerns can be addressed and documented early in the illness, this can reassure patients and carers that their wishes will be respected. It enables them to "retain a voice" when their own voice is weak. One can imagine the individual's frustration knowing that other people are making decisions on their behalf, contrary to their wishes when they still have capacity but have difficulty expressing those wishes verbally.

> He always said to me that once he was unable to swallow he didn't want anything to prolong his life. He always loved his food but didn't want a tube in his stomach. Unfortunately the doctors thought it was the best thing to do as his swallowing was unsafe and he was unable to tell them what he wanted now. I wish they had asked me first. (Sister of a 76-year-old man with advanced Parkinson's disease)

Unfortunately, some people wrongly assume that just because a person has slow or difficult speech, they also have impairment of their cognitive function. There can be a temptation to finish the person's sentence for them or guess what they are trying to say in an attempt to help them; this can be frustrating and patronizing for that individual. Individuals may be excluded from discussions and talked over because others have incorrectly assumed they have lost capacity.

Range of Speech Problems

Speech problems can take various forms. In those who have experienced a stroke, there may be dysphasia (difficulty finding the words mentally) or dysarthria (knowing the words but having difficulty expressing them clearly and intelligibly), depending on which areas of the brain have been affected. Dysphasia can involve both the understanding of speech (receptive dysphasia) and the production of speech (expressive dysphasia). This is the most common language disorder cause by stroke [4]. In the case of expressive dysphasia, an individual may understand exactly what someone is saying to them but cannot communicate their response in return. Alternatively, in the case of receptive dysphasia, they may have fluent comprehensible speech, but it becomes apparent they do not understand what is said as their responses are incongruent with what is being asked of them. Dysarthria is a problem only with the muscles involved in the production of speech which makes the speech sound different. There is no problem with comprehension or the content of the speech.

Dyspraxia is a problem with coordination of speech when the individual muscles used to produce speech are not weakened or damaged, but the control of them is incorrect. This may result in mispronunciation or incorrect order of words.

Many patients with Parkinson's disease will have speech problems when they first develop the condition, and up to 50 % will develop problems with speech and communication at some point in the illness [5]. This may take the form of slow, quiet, monotonous speech or hoarse, unsteady speech. In a similar way to the difficulties with starting walking, some patients may find it difficult to start a conversation and then find they are talking faster and faster without control as the speech starts to flow.

Multiple sclerosis (MS) can cause what is sometimes described as "staccato" jerky speech or dysarthric speech with imprecise pronunciation of vowels and consonants. The prevalence of dysarthria in MS is reported as being between 25 % and 55 % [3]. There may be a nasal quality to the speech due to inability to control the flow of air through the nose while talking. They may also demonstrate excess variation in pitch and volume of their voice as a result of poor breathing control.

> When we started to notice my speech was getting difficult we spoke with the doctor and specialist nurse and they helped us to make a plan about what I wanted to happen as my condition deteriorated. My family and I found this very helpful and I continued to feel in control of what happened to me even when I couldn't get the words out. I carry the form with me and show it to all the doctors and nurses when I go to hospital. (40-year-old lady with speech impairment secondary to MS who completed a "preferred priorities for care" document)

> I can't control what is happening with the disease but I can control what happens to me. (39-year-old man with progressive MS)

When advance care planning discussions are initiated early in the journey, the outcome of this process can be highly successful for the patient and satisfying for the professionals involved. A great deal can be learned from these discussions which can help to build rapport and understanding between all concerned. It may be difficult to raise the idea of planning for anticipated deterioration. Yet, there are tangible benefits for the patient if this is done with appropriate training and compassion and will usually outweigh any concern over causing unnecessary distress. The correct time to raise these issues will vary from individual to individual, depending on their symptoms, their mental capacity, and whether they are someone who likes to talk about the future. It can be difficult to recognize when someone with a neurological condition is reaching the end of life phase, but there are certain "triggers" [6] which can help to recognize this phase – see Chap. 2.

Cognitive Problems

Cognitive change is frequently seen within the spectrum of neurological disease and yet seldom discussed and planned for in advance.

The severity of cognitive change will vary between the different neurological conditions and also between individuals with the same condition. However, lack of information, advance planning, and discussion can cause unnecessary additional distress and anxiety to families, who are not prepared for the cognitive changes and how to manage them. Cognitive problems which are not anticipated can be particularly distressing to the family if they happen when the patient is approaching the transition to end of life care.

The Impact of Cognitive Change

The word "cognition" relates to the higher functions of the brain. This includes the mental processes of language, memory, perception, and executive functioning. Executive functions are those which allow us to connect past experience to present action, for example, anticipating that a weakness of the right hand may not improve and then being able to change future behavior to account for this. Cognitive change can vary, occasionally improving, although progression is more common. It can take many forms including impulsive behavior or aggression. Some patients become obsessive, while others may show emotional lability or confusion.

The assessment and successful management of cognitive change are vitally important because they can alter many areas of an individual's life. Some individuals may no longer be able to continue working in the same job using the same equipment. Some people may experience problems maintaining the physical and emotional relationship with their loved ones. Cognitive changes may affect the individual's ability to adapt to the illness and retain some independence by driving a car or using a telephone for communication.

A change in a person's cognition can also have profound effects on those caring for them. Carers may notice that the patient is unable to do more than one task at once and has difficulty with concentration or word-finding problems. These simple changes can develop into more complex problems including not being able to plan ahead regarding finances or weigh up the benefits and risks of a treatment or procedure. It may prove particularly difficult to weigh up the options during end of life care when there is cognitive impairment.

Cognitive changes can be a significant barrier to effective communication both with families or carers and the health professionals involved in their care. Discussions about future care and planning around end of life care can be difficult regardless of whether there is cognitive change and are therefore sometimes avoided by both patients and professionals. All too often, important discussions about advance care planning are triggered only when cognitive impairment is well established, and then, it may be too late to involve the patient fully as they have lost capacity to participate in these more complex decisions. The issue of cognitive impairment needs to be raised early in the disease process so that patients, carers, and other professionals involved can be fully involved in decision-making before capacity to do so is lost. Advance care planning is not an outcome but a process. It should ideally take place over a period of time as professionals get to know the individual and can help to discuss and document the patient's concerns and wishes for the future. These discussions can be held with any professional involved in the care. Further discussion about advance care planning can be found in Chap. 7.

> They tried to ask her what she wanted to happen at the end. But by that point she had trouble remembering who I was let alone the choices the doctor had just said to her. Instead they asked me what I thought she would want. We hadn't talked about it because we didn't know what was coming but I think I know what she would have wanted. (Husband of a 73-year-old lady who had suffered a severe stroke)

Mental Capacity Assessment

The mental capacity of a person is the mental ability to make a particular decision or take a particular action for themselves. It is important to note that this can fluctuate, and a decision may need to be delayed if it is expected that capacity will be subsequently resumed, for example, after treatment of a urinary tract infection which has caused acute confusion. Further discussion about capacity can be found in Chap. 7, but it is important to mention that there should be an assumption that a patient has capacity until proven otherwise with formal testing (see Table 3.1).

If cognitive deterioration is likely, a patient's wishes can be heard before they lose capacity. Mechanisms such as appointing a lasting power of attorney for health and social welfare (LPA) can give the individual the important reassurance that decisions will not be made for them without consultation with the LPA. Decisions where an LPA could be involved might be whether to insert a feeding tube in someone with MND who had lost capacity at the time. In practice, treatments and procedures can happen because the team feels it is the best interest decision for the patient. However, the individual may have communicated earlier in the illness that they

Table 3.1 Capacity questions

To test if the person has capacity
Does the person have an impairment of the mind or brain or a disturbance of mental function?
If so, does that impairment or disturbance mean that the person is unable to make the decision in question at the time it needs to be made?
To have capacity to make a decision someone must be able to
Understand the information relevant to the decision
Retain the information
Use that information as part of the process of making the decision
Communicate his/her decision either by talking, signing, or any other means

Adapted from http://www.patient.co.uk/doctor/Mental-Capacity-Act.htm

would not want their life prolonged with a feeding tube, even though this may result in shortening their life.

Family and friends may notice the changes in cognition but not fully understand that this may be related to the underlying disease process. There may be a fear that the individual is suffering from another condition such as Alzheimer's disease or a brain tumor, and then the family experience almost relief when they discover it is part of the same disease spectrum.

> This must sound strange to you but I feel so relieved that his memory problems are part of the Parkinson's disease. I was afraid that he had a brain tumour and we just couldn't cope with another problem as big as that. (Wife and carer of a man with advanced Parkinson's disease)

It is important to assess the presence of cognitive change as early as possible after symptoms are recognized and identify ways to help those affected. Within each progressive neurological disease, there are cognitive impairment changes which may be characteristic of that disease. However, regardless of the underlying condition, it is worth noting that an individual may demonstrate significant behavioral and cognitive change as a direct result of the losses and changes he or she has endured. The stigma of a movement disorder or the loss of a job can all contribute to frustration and emotional outbursts, and a lack of emotional control can then result in aggressive behavior toward others.

> He becomes angry at times and can take it out on me. I don't mind though as I understand what he is going through. He was a marathon runner and always kept himself fit. He feels so frustrated that he can no longer walk or feed himself. The doctors thought he might have mild dementia but I think he is just grieving for the life he had. (Wife of a 56-year-old man with limb onset MND)

Coping with Communication Problems

Asking Difficult Questions

Conversations about end of life decisions can be challenging. Asking what people feel and what they want can feel uncomfortable and daunting. In people with neurological conditions, the challenge can be made all the greater in the presence of communication problems. The careful use of questions can help people express themselves. Open questions or prompts which neither direct nor restrict an answer can be most valuable in understanding the person, their priorities, and preferences.

- Useful questions to ascertain what is important to the individual
- "What would you like to see happen from here?"
- "Can you tell me what you understand about what's been happening to you?"
- "Is life still sweet?"
- "What's most important to you right now?"
- "Are you able to say what is worrying you?"

A useful technique is to pick up on cues or events to trigger discussion about end of life wishes, for example, the patient who mentions listening to a program on the radio about euthanasia or who was unhappy about being admitted to hospital.

> You've told me that you felt distressed in hospital. It makes me wonder if we should talk about what you would or wouldn't want to happen should you become less well? There may come a time when it is very difficult for you to communicate at all. It would be helpful for us all if we could know what your wishes are so we can protect you. Would you be willing to talk with us about what you want in the future?

When the end of life is near in neurological diseases, speech can be lost, and only "yes" or "no" may be signaled. Harry's story at the beginning of this chapter demonstrates how the careful use of closed questions can allow the person to continue to control what is happening to them and to communicate any important concerns and wishes as they face their death.

Discussing the Initial Diagnosis of a Neurological Disease

Conveying the diagnosis of a potentially serious neurological disease can be difficult [7]. At diagnosis, the patient and family are embarking on a lifelong relationship with services to support them in their future care, including at the end of life. The development of trust, respect, and security in the person's relationship with health services can be established at this time.

Receiving a diagnosis of a neurological condition is unavoidably disturbing. Even when communication is at its best, reactions to bad news may be challenging. However, in many cases, there is a feeling of relief at finally knowing what is wrong.

> To be honest it was actually a relief to finally get the diagnosis. I know there's been something wrong with me for years. I kept being told it was stress. (47-year-old woman with MS)

Some patients have lived with changes and symptoms for years and have passed through a plethora of medical specialities before final reaching a diagnosis. For others, the diagnosis comes swiftly after the onset of symptoms. Some feel shock as the current symptoms seem insignificant compared to the consequence of the diagnosis.

> I thought he (Consultant Neurologist) was going to tell me I had a slipped disc. (65-year-old woman diagnosed with MND)

Table 3.2 Key tips in giving diagnosis

Basic principles of discussing diagnosis
Invite the person to bring someone with them when they are getting test results
Ensure a private room is available and free from distractions and interruptions
Convey the diagnosis sensitively and at a pace that is manageable for the individual
Allow time for crucial information to sink in
Avoid medical jargon
Keep checking that the individual understands what has been said. For example, ask open questions to gauge their level of understanding
Immediate support after diagnosis
Offer literature about their disease to read later
Provide a follow-up contact number
Arrange a review appointment in the near future for further discussion
Provide information about sources of condition specific and general support
Provide a quiet room or other similar facility, where they may rest before they leave
Start difficult discussions at or soon after diagnosis by exploring people's attitudes and views before decisions have to be made and any possible cognitive change has developed

For the majority of people, they know that something is far from right, and often their fears are confirmed when the diagnosis is finally reached.

Giving the diagnosis requires great sensitivity from the clinician including listening to the patient's understanding of what has been said and any questions they have. Sadly, the giving of a difficult diagnosis is often not well handled and can leave a sense of mistrust and isolation for the patient. Clinicians admit their own inadequacies and strategies to avoid difficult conversations.

> I tell them I'm referring them onto a regional specialist for a second opinion…that usually stops them asking me too much.

> The good news about MND (motor neurone disease) is that it doesn't cause pain or bladder problems.

The environment and support immediately after the giving of a diagnosis can have a lasting impact on the patient's experience.

> I was devastated. I walked out of the clinic room with my head swimming. I wanted to break down and cry, but I had to walk down a long corridor with people sitting along both sides. I felt that they were all staring at me, it was awful. I will never ever forget that day. (65-year-old woman with MND)

There are some basic guiding principles which can help when discussing a new diagnosis (see Table 3.2)

Planning for Changes in Communication

Changes in communication can often be anticipated. Early changes in communication should trigger preparation for the future and the involvement of a speech and language therapist. Acknowledging that communication is likely to get worse can be a difficult discussion. Some patients and their family find reassurance in knowing that help is available and being able to plan for their future. Early changes in speech are a prompt to explore end of life wishes with the patient, including consideration of an advanced directive or appointment of a lasting power of attorney. Early planning in response to speech changes should also focus on developing practical coping strategies.

The creation of a life storybook or other similar biographical record before communication becomes difficult will be helpful to some people. These records can be a powerful tool for self-expression when other means of communication may be lost. A life storybook can encourage health-care staff to see beyond the illness and understand the person [8, 9]

When loss of speech is expected, patients should consider digitally recording their own voices. This might include words or phrases that could be incorporated in a communication device at a later date [10]

Coping with Speech Changes

Changes in speech due to dysarthria will commonly worsen over time in progressive neurological conditions. In some conditions, for example, motor neuron disease, the speed of change can be rapid. Understanding and anticipating speech changes can help the patient and family to adapt and successfully adopt coping strategies [11]. Methods to supplement or replace speech are known as augmentative and alternative communication (AAC). These methods range from simple unaided techniques, such as signing and body language through to high technology using computers and speech-generating systems.

Involvement of a speech and language therapist is important in planning and implementing appropriate AAC. Ongoing assessment of the patient's capability, including cognitive impairment, will guide choice of methods recommended. Cognitive limitations are the primary reason for rejection of ACC technology [11].

Unaided forms of ACC include those which require no external tool and include simple methods such as facial expression, sign language, and gestures. These methods can be part of our natural communication repertoire, are possible for most patients to use, and are easily understood by attentive listeners. A simple smile and nod can convey much in a conversation.

Harry's story at the beginning of this chapter illustrates that at the very end of life, communication can be limited to communicating a simple "yes" or "no" through a blink, squeeze, or other consistent means of signaling. The use of careful explanation and closed questions can allow important communication to continue despite profound disability.

Aided forms of ACC include use of external tools to aid communication and range from the simple to complex technological devices. Simple tools can include writing and communication boards. For some patients, with bulbar forms of MND, for example, writing with pen and paper is preferred as this allows quick and

Fig 3.1 A simple communication board

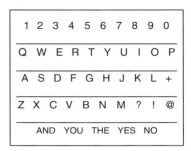

1	2	3	4	5	6	7	8	9	0
Q	W	E	R	T	Y	U	I	O	P
A	S	D	F	G	H	J	K	L	+
Z	X	C	V	B	N	M	?	!	@
AND	YOU	THE	YES	NO					

Fig 3.2 A Lightwriter®
electronic speech generating
system

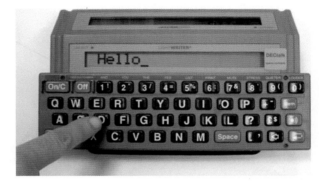

unlimited expression. In the case of hypophonia, for example, in Parkinson's disease, the use of a simple voice amplifier can be helpful.

Communication boards can be an invaluable tool to aid communication. An alphabet board can be used for spelling out words. These boards can be used to supplement verbal communication in the spelling of words proving difficult to say or hear. In cases of loss of speech, communication boards can be the main method of communication. Bespoke communication boards can be made to the individual's needs and capability, for example, a board with frequent requests or a board with pictures of activities or emotions if a person may understand pictures better than words. Patients can indicate the required image through pointing or eye gaze, or they may indicate yes or no as the listener points at the images. Creating a bespoke communication board can be a means of imparting a sense of control back to the patient and respect for their need to express themselves.

See Fig. 3.1

Complex aided AAC tools include electronic speech-generating systems. Commonly used devices in the UK are the Lightwriter®, a keyboard system which will speak the text as typed, and the Apple iPad, or other tablet computers with speech production apps. The systems can be programmed with common phrases and can predict text as typed. In the case of people with progressive neurological conditions, these tools tend to be used by patients with good cognitive ability and dexterity. More sensitive electronic speech generation systems are available, including those which track eye movements to indicate a word or phrase.

See Fig. 3.2

Table 3.3 Key tips for coping with dysarthria

Minimize background noise and distractions
Establish clear signals for "yes" and "no"
Ask the person if there is anything important they would like to talk about
Check that you have heard correctly "Can I just check that I've understood…"
Do not pretend you have understood
Avoiding rushing to assume what is being said
Ask the person to spell out any difficult words
Encourage the person to slow down and take breaths between words
Seek permission to include family members who may be more able to understand
If understanding is not possible, then apologize and offer time to rest and to return later

To be successful in people with progressive neurological conditions, communication aids or strategies need to be introduced early [12]. The use of a communication device can restore the ability to communicate, and this has been shown to have a great effect on quality of life [13]. Advice can be given both to patients and carers which can help them to cope with the dysarthria (see Table 3.3)

Communication: Coping with Cognitive Problems

Communication is our means of expression. The loss of language skills in cognitive impairment can coincide with the development of unusual behaviors and repeated confused ideas or questions. These can be a sign of a need to express something, sometimes real worries. The cornerstone of communication in cognitive changes is to understand the nature of these changes and to interpret nonverbal communication and changes in behavior.

Tension and conflict can develop when cognitive changes occur. It may be helpful to explore cognitive changes openly with the patient and loved ones. Some reassurance and relief may be found from understanding why changes have occurred.

> I didn't realise MS could affect my mind, I thought I was getting Alzheimer's as well! (Patient with MS and memory problems)

Open conversations about cognitive issues may not be acceptable or possible. Such consultations can exacerbate conflict if a patient is unable to acknowledge there is a problem. Support for carers is vital to help their coping. This support should focus on understanding the nature of cognitive problems and advice on strategies to cope and aid communication (see Table 3.4)

Carers of people with cognitive problems often report not knowing how to deal with difficult cognitive issues affecting communication [14]. Finding the balance between confronting and colluding is an ongoing dilemma. In most cases, the balance depends on the situation and context.

The repeat of a common confusion may give useful insight into real fears or worries

> He keeps on and on about having to get to a conference and that he's waiting for faxes to come through about tyres. I keep telling him he's confused and he doesn't need to worry about anything. (Wife of patient with advanced MS. Patient previously had a tire business)

Table 3.4 Key tips for coping with communication issues in cognitive impairment

Respect for person
Always include the person in conversations even if little or no response
Introduce yourself each time and ask permission to speak with them
Getting to know the person can help in predicting worries or reactions
Confused thinking
Avoid agreeing with confused ideas, but be flexible
Use distraction and diversion onto another topic
Focus on feelings rather than facts
Listening skills
Help the person to find other ways of saying what they want to if struggling to find words
Paraphrase what you have heard to check if you have understood correctly
Speaking clearly
Use simple, short sentences
Avoid direct or complex questions.
If questions are necessary, use simple closed questions allowing a "yes" or "no" answer
Try different ways of saying the same thing, if not being understood despite repeating
Patience
Allow time for person to process information and to respond

Adapted from *Coping with Dementia: A Practical Handbook for Carers* (2009) and Alzheimer's Society Communication Factsheet

Through discussion with this patient and his family, it became clear that he had a strong sense of his role as provider and he previously had a tight control over the tire business and household money. He was genuinely worried about their financial security and felt impotent to influence how their money was being managed. His family had felt it was kinder to tell him not to worry. This had the effect of increasing his anxiety and frustration when he was unable to clearly express his worries. Time spent as a family going through bank statements and meeting with their accountant did help relieve some fears. The family no longer dismisses his concerns; they give time to repeat reassuring information about their finances, including a letter from their accountant. Although he still talks of attending to business, there is less anxiety, and he dwells less on the issue.

Understanding Distress in People with Communication and Cognitive Problems

Patients with cognitive impairment are less likely to be treated for pain and depression [15, 16]. While tools are available to help understand if a person is in distress, it is often more difficult to understand the cause of any distress.

> Patient with Parkinson's disease and dementia looking anxiously over the nurse's shoulder.
> Patient: "Tell them to stop hitting my lump."
> Nurse: "What's being hit?"
> Patient: "They're hitting my lump."

Table 3.5 Signs of pain in people with cognitive or communication impairment

Type	Description
Autonomic changes	Pallor, sweating, tachypnea, altered breathing patterns, tachycardia, hypertension
Facial expressions	Grimacing, wincing, frowning, rapid blinking, brow raising, brow lowering, cheek raising, eyelid tightening, nose wrinkling, lip corner pulling, chin raising, lip puckering
Body movements	Altered gait, pacing, rocking, hand wringing, repetitive movements, increased tone, guarding,[a] bracing[b]
Verbalizations	Sighing, grunting, groaning, moaning, screaming, calling out, aggressive/ offensive speech
Interpersonal interactions	Aggression, withdrawal, resisting
Activity patterns	Wandering, altered sleep, altered rest patterns
Mental status changes	Confusion, crying, distress, irritability

RCP (2007), Royal College of Physicians
[a]Guarding = "abnormal stiff, rigid, or interrupted movement while changing position"
[b]Bracing = a stationary position in which a fully extended limb maintains and supports an abnormal weight distribution for at least 3 s

> Nurse: "Do you mean your knee, here?"
> Nurse gently placing her hand on knee of patient's contracted leg.
> Patient: "Yes, they're hitting that lump."

This patient's regular analgesia had been discontinued as care home staff reported he was not in pain. He was known to hallucinate, and this regular comment was dismissed as meaningless confusion. His leg was bent in fixed flexion at his knee such that all he might see or feel of his lower leg would in effect be a lump. It was very possible that he was experiencing a thumping pain in this knee. This simple conversation was the prompt for a multidisciplinary review of his pain, spasticity, and positioning. It is always helpful and sometimes enlightening to try and see the world from the patient's perspective. People with cognitive problems may struggle to explain their experience in an expected way. This technique can offer logical explanations for what may at first seem confused nonsense. "Distress may be hidden, but is rarely silent." [15] (See Table 3.5)

End of Life Decisions and Cognitive Problems

Important issues related to end of life decisions ideally should be explored before cognitive problems progress. In reality, the triggers for these important discussions often come later in the disease progression when the person may no longer have mental capacity to consider the issues involved. Rarely have people made a formal expression of what their end of life wishes are prior to the onset of significant cognitive problems.

Piecing together a picture of that person's values and beliefs through discussion with those close to them can help us to inform best interest decisions.

> He was a very proud and private man. He wouldn't like the idea of being messed around with, he would hate the indignity of it all. (Daughter of patient with advanced Huntington's disease)

> She's always been a fighter. She never wanted to let MS beat her. I think she still enjoys life, but it's much harder now. She hardly ever gets out now and none of her old friends visit. (Sister of patient with MS)

An understanding of how the condition has progressed and how life has changed for that person and of their pleasure in life can help best interest decisions to be taken.

The involvement of patients with cognitive problems in advance care planning is important. This will be limited to imparting information rather than involvement in the complex decisions. Complicated concepts and questions may cause bewilderment, insecurity, and distress for the cognitively impaired patient. The use of carefully planned communication skills to inform the patient of what is happening to them may reduce distress and aid coping.

Conclusion

In the more advanced stages of neurological disease, patients often become more aware that nothing will alter the course of the disease. When neurological disease advances and disability increases, access to specialist clinical care can become more difficult. Some clinicians readily identify their own feelings of powerlessness to know how to help, but those of us who are privileged to work routinely with these people will instinctively recognize the individual behind the disease. With all the potential problems of speech difficulties and even in progressive cognitive change, people have a real human need to communicate, to express themselves. The essence of good communication in neurological disease is to seek out and communicate, somehow, with the person behind their disease.

References

1. Brown C. My left foot. London: Vintage; 1998. p. p17.
2. Bolmsjo I. Existential issues in palliative care: interviews of patients with amyotrophic lateral sclerosis. J Palliat Med. 2001;4(2):499–505.
3. Talking about communication in multiple sclerosis, information sheet. Rehabilitation in multiple sclerosis. Milan: RIMS Publications; 3, 2007.
4. Cognitive problems after stroke, factsheet 7. The stroke association. www.stroke.org.uk. Accessed on 25 July 2011.

5. Speech and Language Therapy information sheet. Parkinson's Disease Society. http://www.parkinsons.org.uk/. Accessed on 25 July 2011.
6. NHS National End of Life Care Programme. Improving end of life care in neurological disease. Executive summary. 2010.
7. National End of Life Care Programme, National Council for Palliative Care, The Neurological Alliance. Improving end of life care in neurological disease: a framework for implementation. Leicester: NHS National End of Life Care Programme; 2010.
8. Mckeown J, Clarke A, Repper J. Life story work in health and social care: systematic literature review. J Adv Nurs. 2006;55(2):237–47.
9. Wills T, Day MR. Valuing the person's story: use of life story books in a continuing care setting. Clin Interv Aging. 2008;3(3):547–52.
10. Singleton E, Rosenfeld J. Voice banking to facilitate compliance with speech generating augmentative communication. Amyotroph Lateral Scler. 2010;11(42):1748–2968.
11. Ball LJ, Beukelman DR, Pattee GL. Acceptance of augmentative and alternative communication technology by persons with amytrophic lateral sclerosis. Augment Altern Commun. 2004;20(2):113–22.
12. Doyle M, Philips B. Trends in augmentative and alternative communication use by individuals with amyotrophic lateral sclerosis. Augment Altern Commun. 2001;17(3):167–78.
13. Schmalbach S, Sieniawski M, Kollewe K, Dengler R, Krampfl K, Petri S, Sieniawski M, Kollewe K, Dengler R, Krampfl K, Petri S. Speech therapy and communication devices: impact on quality of life in patients with ALS. Amyotroph Lateral Scler. 2010;11(132): 1748–2968.
14. Hasson F, Kernohan WG, McLaughlin M, Waldron M, McLaughlin D, Chambers H, Cochrane B. An exploration into the palliative and and-of-life experiences of carers of people with Parkinson's disease. Palliat Med. 2010;24(7):731–6.
15. Regnard C, Reynolds J, Watson B, Matthews D, Gibson L, Clarke C. Understanding distress in people with severe communication difficulties. J Intellect Disabil Res. 2007;51(4):277–92.
16. Van Iersel T, Timmerman D, Mullie A. Introduction of a pain scale for palliative care patients with cognitive impairment. Int J Palliat Nurs. 2006;12(2):54–9.

Chapter 4
Physical Symptoms in Neurological Conditions

Mark Lee

Abstract Physical symptoms are a common problem in all progressive neurological conditions and can occur at any stage of disease. These symptoms are optimally treated through a combination of careful patient-centered assessment, timely intervention, open and honest discussion, realistic goal setting, planning ahead, coordination of care, and regular review of patient and carer.

This chapter will consider the wider context for treating physical symptoms, the principles for their assessment, and the role of the management of the underlying neurological condition. Specific symptoms will be discussed in terms of their prevalence, mechanisms, and treatments. These will be explored under the headings:

1. Physical symptoms which are common to a number of neurological conditions (e.g., breathlessness, pain, sleep disorders)
2. The management of symptoms which are specific to particular neurological conditions

The neurological diseases discussed in this chapter are multiple sclerosis (MS), Parkinson's disease (PD), progressive supranuclear palsy (PSP), multiple system atrophy (MSA), motor neuron disease (MND), Huntington's disease (HD), and stroke disease.

Keywords Assessment • Symptom • Neurological • Multidisciplinary • Patient factors

M. Lee, MBChB, MRCP, M.D.
Department of Palliative Care, St. Benedict's Hospice & City Hospitals,
Newcastle Road, Sunderland, Tyne and Wear SR5 1NB, UK
e-mail: mark.lee@sotw.nhs.uk

D. Oliver (ed.), *End of Life Care in Neurological Disease*,
DOI 10.1007/978-0-85729-682-5_4, © Springer-Verlag London 2013

Case Study

Mr. A was a 70-year gentleman who was referred from neurology to the palliative care outpatient clinic with a 14-year history of Parkinson's disease. In those years, he was treated with procyclidine (antimuscarinic), selegiline/rasagiline (monoamine oxidase B inhibitor), bromocriptine/cabergoline (dopamine agonists), co-beneldopa (levodopa), and entacapone (catechol-O-methyltransferase inhibitor). Under the care of the neurology team, his drug regime had settled to Madopar five tablets a day, Sinemet CR 125 mg at night, and selegiline once daily. Over the 14 years, he had developed complications of dopaminergic therapy becoming increasingly immobile and increasingly dependent on his wife for his activities of daily living.

He had always been an active man who enjoyed writing, drawing, and playing the piano. However, the progression of his disease had severely affected his ability to do these and had understandably become a source of frustration. He was bradykinetic, tremulous, and had difficulty speaking.

He remained under neurology review. He also had continued input from physiotherapists, occupational therapists, and speech and language therapists (SALT).

He had developed nocturia and bladder spasm over the last few years. In the last year, he had had multiple admissions to hospital. Initially, his symptoms were attributed to outflow obstruction and settled following a transurethral resection of prostate (TURP) and later by insertion of a suprapubic catheter. He developed further bladder spasms which were controlled in part with antimuscarinic drugs, but there also seemed to be relief provided on occasions by dispersible Madopar. As the pain became more resistant to these treatments, he found benefit with low-dose opioids (immediate-release morphine). His chronic constipation was controlled with oral laxatives although enemas were sometimes required.

Mr. A also had problems with drooling and often had to change his shirts. There were no obvious reversible factors causing the drooling, so he was commenced on a hyoscine hydrobromide patch every 3 days. This was only partially effective, so he was switched to glycopyrronium solution with good effect.

His speech and swallowing continued to deteriorate over the next 12 months. He was also showing signs of cognitive impairment. His speech was difficult to understand, he had poor oral intake, his weight was dropping, and he was becoming increasingly immobile. After multidisciplinary discussion involving SALT, dietitian, gastroenterologist, neurologist, him, and his wife, a percutaneous endoscopic gastrostomy (PEG) was inserted, and following a prolonged admission to hospital, he was discharged to a care home in order to optimally meet his nursing needs.

He then suffered recurrent urinary tract and chest infections, all of which worsened his condition. These were treated after discussion with his family and provided good symptomatic relief. Wider discussions about his deteriorating condition continued and were acknowledged by family and health-care professionals.

Three years after the initial referral to the specialist palliative care service and 17 years after his diagnosis of Parkinson's disease, he died peacefully in the care home with his family by his bed.

The Context for Treating Physical Symptom

The case of Mr. A illustrates the complex and dynamic context in which physical symptoms can occur in patients with long-term neurological conditions. Therefore, before looking at specific physical symptoms, we need to understand more of this wider context. We will look briefly at:

- Patient factors
- Carer factors
- Health-care factors
- Limited evidence base

Patient Factors

These aspects may affect the assessment of and treatment options available for any particular symptom:

- The progressive nature of the neurological condition
- The rate and unpredictability of this progression
- The degree of disability at the time of assessment
- The presence of neuropsychiatric symptoms (such as cognitive impairment, hallucinations, or depression) and their effect on the patients' decision-making capacity

The overall symptom burden may also be important. For example, some patients may describe one or two dominant symptoms, while others describe a large number of smaller more irritating symptoms. A study in Parkinson's disease (PD) demonstrated that the mean number of symptoms in patients at all stages of disease was 14.3 (median 14, range 0–29) [1]. A further study in PD patients (mean age$=70\pm$ 8.6 years) highlighted the frequency of comorbid diseases in this group with 84 % having one or more moderate comorbid condition and 15 % having a severe comorbidity [2]. Significant numbers of comorbid conditions are also present in other neurological conditions [3, 4]. These themselves may be responsible for significant or even dominating symptoms in neurological conditions. In this context, early holistic assessment, patient-led prioritizing, realistic goal setting, and liaison with other specialties are vital in order to meaningfully reduce the symptom burden and help future planning.

Carer Factors

A UK survey of over 3,000 carers of patients with Parkinson's disease in 2007 demonstrated that 27 % had been caring for over 10 years, 63 % spent more than 50 h a week looking after their relative, and over 50 % felt their physical and mental health had deteriorated since caring [5]. Other progressive neurological conditions show similar affects on carers [6]. Support for carers themselves is therefore crucial – see Chap. 9. Furthermore, in this stressful context, relatively mild physical symptoms or chronic intractable symptoms can become a "tipping point" in the patients' care.

Health-Care Factors

National guidance has highlighted the patchy nature of service provision for patients with long-term neurological conditions in the UK [7]. It has also highlighted the need for communication and coordination of existing services [8]. The case of Mr. A aptly demonstrates that many specialists and allied health-care professionals often need to be involved in a patient's care. The role of primary care, social workers, and voluntary agencies can also not be overestimated. Good symptom control in this context may well be determined by not only the availability of local services but also the coordination of and communication between those services which do exist. The use of a nominated key worker to coordinate this process (such as the specialist neurology nurse) is therefore important.

These national publications also highlight the need for workforce development in the care of patients with long-term neurological conditions. A survey of neurology nurses in 2008 revealed that over 70 % of respondents felt they had palliative care training needs and over 40 % felt that these were in the area of symptom control [9].

Limited Evidence Base

There are very few good-quality randomized control trials looking at treating symptoms in progressive neurological conditions. On the other hand, some commonly used treatments have been extrapolated from studies in other diseases (such as opioids for breathlessness) or have become "best practice" after years of clinical experience (e.g., hyoscine hydrobromide patches for drooling). Therefore, the nature of the current evidence and the need for further more robust studies mean that any recommendations of a particular treatment will be necessarily tentative.

Table 4.1 The range of symptoms reported in four neurological conditions (symptoms are listed alphabetically not in order of frequency)

MND	MS	PD	PSP
Ankle edema	Ataxia	Anorexia	Bradykinesia
Chest infection	Bladder issues	Bradykinesia	Dysarthria
Constipation	Bowel issues	Constipation	Dysphagia
Drooling	Contractures	Drooling	Dysphonia
Dysarthria	Dysarthria	Drowsiness	Dystonia
Dysphagia	Dysphagia	Dry mouth	Falls
Dyspnea	Fatigue	Dyspnea	Fatigue
Immobility	Immobility	Hallucinations	Incontinence
Incontinence	Pain	Immobility	Muscle pain
Insomnia	Pressure sores	Insomnia	Tremor
Pain	Sexual issues	Nausea	Visual issues
Pressure sores	Spasticity	Pain	
Vomiting	Tremor	Stiffness/rigidity	
Weakness	Weakness	Tremor	
Weight loss		Vivid dreams	

Physical Symptoms and Their Assessment

Symptoms

There are a wide range of physical symptoms in progressive neurological conditions, and they can affect multiple body systems. Table 4.1 shows examples of some of the symptoms which have been reported in published literature for different diseases (MND [10, 11], MS [12], PD [1, 13], PSP [14, 15]). The lists are by no means exhaustive but do illustrate that they tend to fall into two main groups:

- Symptoms which are common to a number of neurological conditions (e.g., pain, dysarthria, incontinence, and immobility)
- Symptoms which are more often observed in specific diseases (e.g., ataxia in MS and visual problems in PSP)

The number and prevalence of symptoms found in neurological conditions are comparable to those found in cancer patients [1].

Assessment

We have already considered the wider context in which physical symptoms in neurological conditions occur, and as such, the assessment of these symptoms necessarily involves a broad approach. The World Health Organization definition of palliative care promoted this approach to improve quality of life of patients and their families "through the prevention and relief of suffering by means of early identification and impeccable assessment and treatment of pain and other problems, physical, psychosocial and spiritual" [16]. The National Service Framework for Long-term Conditions (UK) has endorsed this approach for patients with neurodegenerative diseases and sets out quality requirements that promote patient-centered care, support for family and carers, multidisciplinary team working, workforce development, and access to palliative care. They highlight, however, that this palliative care approach is not just delivered by specialist palliative care teams but must also be employed by any team which is involved in the patients' care [17].

Treatment of the Underlying Neurological Condition

Treatment of the underlying neurological condition could potentially have a huge effect on relieving the symptom burden on both patients and families.

Preventing Disease Progression Will Have an Impact on the Rate of Symptom Development

The development of therapies in order to slow down or prevent neuron degeneration in neurological conditions is ongoing but to date has largely proved unsuccessful. Currently, there are no known therapies available which have proven to be truly neuroprotective in PD, HD, or MS. However, there have been some treatments in MND, MS, and stroke disease which appear to slow disease progression.

One of the mechanisms postulated for neuronal damage in MND is the accumulation of glutamate. Riluzole reduces the levels of CNS glutamate and has been shown to prolong survival by a median of 2–3 months. The effect on symptoms (e.g., muscle strength) is less clear [18]. The evidence for antioxidants is poor though drugs like vitamin C and E are often used [19].

The primary mechanism in MS is demyelination which in part is thought to be an inflammatory process. As such, many of the drugs which can affect disease progression have an anti-inflammatory or immunomodulatory action. It is beyond the scope of this small section to look in detail at the large number of drugs which have been studied in MS. However, guidelines [12] suggest that there may be roles for several medications, but the relative risks and benefits need to be weighed up with the patient and family under the guidance of an experienced MS team.

Treatments Available for the Condition Which May Help Symptom Control

PD

Motor Symptoms

The cardinal features of PD are bradykinesia (slowness of movement), rigidity, tremor, and postural instability, and from Table 4.1, it can be seen that these are part of the symptom burden in these patients. The control of these symptoms is best achieved through the use of dopaminergic drugs (e.g., levodopa and dopamine agonists), and this can maintain control for a number of years. With longer-term treatment, motor fluctuations appear, such as wearing off and dyskinesia, which necessitate alterations in the drug regime. Drug regimes can become increasingly complex, and the timing of medications is crucial to achieving motor symptom control. In later disease, the dopaminergic response tends to decrease, and patients can find the side effects of treatment more troublesome than the disease itself. Symptom control at this stage can be very challenging and ideally requires liaison with PD specialists.

Evidence suggests that one reason why symptom control in hospital or care homes in PD is suboptimal is due to problems with getting dopaminergic medication on time [20].

Non-motor Symptoms

These symptoms are becoming increasingly recognized as a significant source of morbidity in patients with PD [21]. The range of non-motor symptoms associated with "wearing off" include pain, numbness, chest discomfort, slowness of thinking, hot and cold tolerance, tiredness, restlessness, and bladder difficulties [22]. These symptoms appear to be dopamine responsive in around 50 % of cases in on study (comparable to motor responses) [23].

At all stages, it is important to ensure that dopaminergic treatment is "optimized" as this may help in achieving symptom control. The method used for "optimization" depends on the symptoms expressed, the timing of those symptoms, and the potential drug side effects. Liaison with local PD services is recommended.

MS

Relapsing and remitting MS (RR-MS) is the most common form of MS and, by definition, will have acute episodes or exacerbations of neurological deficits which may or may not completely resolve. However, these episodes have also been described in primary and secondary progressive MS. They are thought to be due to episodes of inflammatory demyelination. Evidence suggests that these relapses should be treated with short-term courses of methylprednisolone (between 3 and 5 days) [24].

Treatment for Physical Symptoms Which Are Common to a Number of Neurological Conditions

Most work has been undertaken in the more common neurodegenerative conditions (i.e., MS and PD), although the results may be applied to other diseases.

Breathlessness

Breathlessness (or dyspnea) is well recognized in MND due to progressive respiratory muscle weakness. However, it has also been demonstrated that respiratory problems can occur in movement disorders (such as PD, PSP, MSA) [25] and in MS [26].

Dyspnea is defined as the "subjective experience of breathing discomfort" and encompasses not just physiological parameters but also psychological, social, and environmental factors [27]. Higher rates of "perceptions of dyspnea" (despite normal lung function) have been described in PD when compared to controls [28].

Multiple pathophysiological mechanisms are involved in the development of breathlessness in neurological conditions. They can be related primarily to the neurological disease (central or peripheral) or to other coexisting factors (e.g., heart or lung disease).

One mechanism common to all the neurodegenerative conditions (especially when advanced) is the risk of pneumonia (both aspiration and hypostatic). In advanced disease, the risk of pneumonia is increased by:

- Dysphagia
- Weight loss and nutritional issues
- Increasing immobility
- Progressive muscle weakness which can diminish the ability to cough and clear bronchial secretions effectively

The treatment of dyspnea will require a broad approach following a full assessment of physical, psychological, social, and environmental aspects.

Management

Nondrug

Physical

- Physiotherapy input can be employed in neurodegenerative conditions in order to improve ventilation and help clear secretions.
- Positional changes, such as sitting upright, can help. Indeed, some patients may need postural aids/supports to maintain an optimum position, especially as the disease progresses.
- In those patients with MND who have an ineffective cough due to respiratory muscle weakness, the use of mechanical insufflation/exsufflation *or* manually assisted cough can be helpful in clearing upper airway secretions [29]. This may be particularly helpful in acute infections.
- A systematic review [30] looking at nondrug interventions for breathlessness, mainly in COPD, demonstrated beneficial effect from:

    - The use of walking aids
    - Neuromuscular electrical stimulation
    - Chest wall vibration
    - Breathing training

- The review did not recommend the use of fans, acupuncture, or relaxation, but they may prove helpful in individual patients.

Psychological

- Exploring anxieties, fears, or panic associated with breathlessness is important.

Drug

- Treat any underlying cause (e.g., infection or airway reversibility).
- Optimize parkinsonian medication in PD.
- Opioids:

    - The precise mechanism of how opioids help breathlessness is unclear; however, a systematic review of their use via the oral or parenteral route to palliate breathlessness (mainly in COPD) demonstrated a significantly positive effect [31].

- Benzodiazepines:

    - The results from a systematic review of the use of benzodiazepines for breathlessness in cancer and COPD reported a slight but nonsignificant trend toward a beneficial effect. They recommended benzodiazepines (such as diazepam or lorazepam) for third-line use after nondrug therapies and opioids [32].

- In refractory cases, mechanical ventilation may be required. This most often occurs in MND patients after multidisciplinary discussions with patient and family (see section "Sleep Disorders").

Constipation

Constipation is very common in all neurodegenerative conditions and may be related to the primary disease or to secondary causes such as existing comorbidities, decreased activity levels, poor fluid intake, and/or medications (levodopa, dopamine agonists, anticholinergics, or opioids). Constipation has been defined by a number of criteria which include symptoms of straining, hard or lumpy stool, sensation of anorectal obstruction, sensation of incomplete evacuation, manual maneuvers to facilitate defecation, and fewer than three defecations per week [33].

The links between the primary neurological disease and constipation have not been fully elucidated; however, a number of mechanisms may be involved, including autonomic dysfunction and altered gut motility.

Management

Nondrug

- Increased dietary fiber/fluid intake
- Increased exercise

Drug

- Review of medications
- Stool softener (e.g., docusate)
- Stool stimulants (e.g., senna or bisacodyl)
- Polyethylene glycol solutions [34]
- Enema or suppositories
- Prokinetics (5HT4 agonists):

    - Prucalopride at doses of 1–4 mg once daily has proved efficacious in elderly patients with chronic constipation [35].
    - Mosapride citrate has also shown positive effects in MSA and PD in case series [36].

Drooling

Drooling is a common problem in neurological disease (e.g., MND = 50–70 % [37], PD = 56 % [38]) and can have a huge negative impact on patients' quality of life.

Normal daily salivary production is between 1 and 1.5 l/day. Drooling is the overflowing of saliva from the mouth and, in the context of neurological disease, may be the result of swallowing dysfunction, excess saliva (or sialorrhea), poor oral control of saliva, or a combination of all three. The evidence in patients with MND [39] suggests that they actually produce decreased amounts of saliva when compared to controls, and therefore, the drooling is thought primarily to be due to dysphagia [40]. In PD, decreased swallowing frequency is also a factor [41].

Management

Nondrug

- Address any underlying cause of increased salivation, such as oral thrush, ill-fitting dentures, or poor oral hygiene.
- Early involvement of speech and language therapy.
- In the context of PD, preliminary work has also been undertaken on a portable metronome broach which alerts at set intervals in order to remind patients to swallow [42].
- Other authors have suggested that chewing gum can also improve the swallow frequency in PD [43].

Drug

Drug therapies for drooling have largely focused on the use of anticholinergics, yet much of the initial data of their efficacy was gained from studies in children with neurodisabilities [44].

- Atropine eye drops given sublingually have shown equivocal results [45].
- Transdermal scopolamine has been shown to be effective for drooling in severely disabled patients [46], but side effects were commonly reported.
- Oral glycopyrrolate (a quaternary amine drug that does not cross the blood-brain barrier) has been shown efficacy in studies in adults with PD [47]. The side effects are generally mild (dry mouth/thick secretions) but may necessitate stopping treatment in some cases.

- Injection of botulinum toxin into the salivary glands can temporarily reduce the volume of saliva between 2 and 6 months. A 2010 international consensus statement concluded that botulinum toxin in adults and children not only improved drooling but had positive impacts on psychosocial aspects of care [48].
- External beam radiotherapy has been used in small studies of MND patients with good effect [49]. Given the irreversible nature of this treatment, it is probably best reserved for refractory cases.

Dysarthria

Dysarthria is defined as difficulty in articulating words and may be a consequence of weakness, incoordination, or spasticity of speech muscles. The social and psychological ramifications of speech difficulties can often be more important than the speech problem itself. Furthermore, the ability to communicate one's wishes is a key part of determining whether a patient has the capacity to make decisions and exercise autonomy.

Dysarthria is common in all neurological conditions (e.g., MND=77 % [50], PD=38–69 % [51]), but the cause of the problem can vary between different diseases. For example, in MND, dysarthria results from weakness or spasticity of the bulbar muscles whereas, in PD, it can result from incoordination of oral and respiratory elements.

In neurodegenerative conditions, dysarthria often coexists with other neurological lesions which can further affect communication. For example:

- Dysphasia (expressive or receptive)
- Bradyphrenia (slow thought processes)
- Cognitive impairment

In advanced disease, communication can be challenging, frustrating, and time consuming for both patients and health-care staff.

Treatment strategies are based on a full assessment of the patient by an experienced speech and language therapist (SALT). Goals and therapies are then tailored to the patients needs.

Management

- Time to speak:

  – As speech slows or quietens, patients with neurological conditions often need more time to express themselves.

- All patients with dysarthria should have a SALT assessment.

  – Exercises:

    Lee Silverman Voice Treatment (LSVT) is one treatment designed for use in PD patients and has been shown to improve voice volume for up to 6 months [52].

  – Augmentative and alternative communication devices:

  Voice amplifiers
  Alphabet boards
  Pacing boards
  Electronic speaking devices (e.g., Lightwriter or iPad).

Dysphagia

Swallowing is a complex neuromuscular process which involves around 50 pairs of muscles and nerves. The overall coordination of the sequential muscle activation is thought to arise from the brainstem [53]. Once activated, there are three phases involved in normal swallowing:

* *The oral phase* – The mouth, through chewing and bolus formation, makes the food or liquid ready for swallowing.
* *The pharyngeal phase* – Begins when the tongue pushes the food or liquid to the back of the mouth. This triggers a swallowing response which passes the bolus through the pharynx while at the same time covering the airway with the epiglottis. This phase is an involuntary reflex.
* *The esophageal phase* – Carries the food bolus from the pharynx to the stomach. This phase is also involuntary, but voluntary swallowing can be triggered from the cerebral cortex.

In neurodegenerative conditions, these phases can be affected even in early disease.

Management

Given the complexity of the deficits in neurodegenerative conditions, the key recommendation in guidelines is early referral to and assessment by an experienced speech and language therapist [12, 54]. Treatments then need to be decided on a case by case basis.

Nondrug

* Speech and language therapy (SALT):

  – In broad terms, the approaches used in SALT are rehabilitative (e.g., post stroke where some recovery may occur), compensatory (where recovery is not likely), or a combination of the two:

  Rehabilitative (or facilitatory) approaches include muscle strengthening exercises and electrical stimulation.
  Compensatory techniques include dietary modification and use of postures/ maneuvers.

Drug

- No drug therapies have been shown to reliably help dysphagia in neurodegenerative conditions; however, in parkinsonian conditions, optimizing levodopa therapy may help in a small number of patients [55].

Enteral Feeding

In patients where there is symptomatic dysphagia with weight loss due to reduced calorie intake, dehydration, or ending meals because of choking, a nasogastric tube (NGT) or percutaneous endoscopic gastrostomy (PEG) might be considered for feeding. The use of NGT or PEG in neurological conditions involves a multidisciplinary assessment and a full discussion with the patient and family. It is seldom a clear-cut decision but rather involves weighing up issues of risks, benefits, autonomy, capacity, culture, prognosis, and expected outcomes.

A systematic review of the use of NGT versus PEG demonstrated that in neurological conditions (mainly stroke) ($n = 109$), PEG had significantly fewer treatment failures. However, in the group as a whole (both neurological and non-neurological), there were no significant differences in mortality rates, complications, or pneumonia. The review suggested that overall survival improved (4.3 months) with PEG use [56].

In MND, some authors suggest that PEG tubes improved nutrition and perhaps prolonged survival, but it is unlikely to prevent aspiration [57].

Nasogastric Tube Feeding

- A role for NGT feeding has been suggested for short-term use, and therefore, it may have more of a role in acute neurological deficits which may recover (e.g., in stroke).
- Short-term use of nasogastric tubes (NGT) has also been suggested in PD in order to deliver dopaminergic medications where there is a temporary loss of swallow. This can be considered when reversible causes (e.g., pneumonia) and an inability to take regular dopaminergic drugs have contributed to the dysphagia.

Percutaneous Endoscopic Gastrostomy

- Recommendations for the use of gastrostomy in MND suggest that an individualized approach should be used looking at the following:

  - Bulbar symptoms
  - Weight loss (>10 %)
  - Patient's overall condition

- It is suggested that in MND, a PEG should be considered early, but if there are increased risks (i.e., FVC <50 % of predicted), then a percutaneous radiologically inserted gastrostomy (PRG) is recommended [57]. A PRG can be placed without any sedation or general anesthetic and is less likely to compromise respiratory function.
- The use of PEGs for nutrition in other neurological conditions has not been clearly defined and hence should be assessed on a case by case basis.
- PEGs and percutaneous endoscopic jejunostomies (PEJ) have been used in advanced PD with success in order to provide continuous infusions of levodopa leading to more stable drug levels and improved motor symptoms [58].

Fatigue

Fatigue is probably one of the most common symptoms experienced by patients with chronic neurological diseases. There is no universally accepted definition of fatigue, and as such, the estimated prevalence in neurological diseases is extremely variable (e.g., MS = 39–78 % [12]). Currently, the causes of fatigue are thought to be multifactorial – some are primarily related to the neurological disease (e.g., disruption of central neural connections [59]) and others to secondary causes (e.g., depression, disability) [60]. Regardless of the cause, it is a symptom which can have a significant negative impact on quality of life.

Management

Nondrug

- Exclude secondary causes of fatigue (e.g., depression).
- Fatigue management such as the use of exercise or of energy conservation/activity pacing is recommended. Good evidence of their efficacy in neurological conditions is lacking.
- In MS, structured "mindfulness-based intervention" has been used in a randomized study with improvements reported for up to 6 months in health-related quality of life, depression, and fatigue [61].

Drug

- Stopping medications which may cause fatigue (e.g., riluzole).
- Fatigue is one of the non-motor symptoms of PD, and as such, optimizing the dopaminergic treatment can help.

- The use of medicines which directly target fatigue should not be used routinely but may be helpful in refractory cases. For example, case series in PD [62] and MS [63] suggest there may be a role for modafinil.

Immobility

The progressive nature of the neurodegenerative conditions means that in many cases mobility will be adversely affected at some point in the disease trajectory. In those conditions where progression is generally slower (e.g., MS, PD, HD, and stroke), there may be opportunities for a rehabilitative approach. In those with more rapidly progressive diseases (e.g., MND) a traditional neurorehabilitative approach is more difficult to apply. However, as one author has stated:

"There are few people with any form of neurological disability who would not benefit from at least some exposure to a team skilled in the basic principles of neurological rehabilitation" [64].

The ramifications of worsening mobility are considerable, and therefore, assessing each of the affected domains is vital in facilitating adjustment to the progressive losses which many patients face. These ramifications include:

- Physical – falls, injury (e.g., fractures), pressure sores, the effect on eliminations, muscle weakness, and inability to carry out activities of daily living
- Psychological – fear, loss of confidence, and loss of independence
- Social – isolation, housebound, and increasing carer strain
- Spiritual – decreased sense of worth, purpose, or meaning
- Environmental – adaptations to home, accepting of external carers, or even a change in care setting

Mobility issues are more common as neurodegenerative diseases progress; however, they often occur at presentation or in early disease. Therefore, *early* assessment by and involvement of specialist multidisciplinary teams are vital first steps in trying to facilitate maximal mobility (and independence) for as long as possible [65].

Management

Recommendations specific for mobility problems in patients with MS provide a useful model with which to approach mobility issues in general in neurological conditions [12].

- Physiotherapy treatments should be offered in order to improve mobility:

  - In parkinsonian disorders, freezing of gait is a common problem being present in around 50 % of patients [66]. Physiotherapy in general and the use of auditory or visual cueing techniques in particular may be helpful [67].

- Consider assessment by a specialist neurological rehabilitation service for:
  - Identification and treatment of the impairment
  - Task-related practice of mobility activities (e.g., transferring)
  - Use of equipment
  - Adaptations to environment
  - Teaching others how to safely help

- Regular reviews are important given the progressive nature of the conditions.
- Planning ahead also needs to be sensitively explored with patients and families.

Pain

Gagliese and Melzack [68] highlighted that pain is a "multidimensional experience with sensory, affective, and cognitive-evaluative components" and, as such, requires a holistic approach to its management. Pain is very common in the general population. In one study, its prevalence in all ages in the community setting was 50 % [69]; however, in elderly patients, pain was present in 70 % [70].

It is on this backdrop that we need to consider the management of pain in neurodegenerative diseases. In particular, our assessment needs to consider not simply the neurological causes of the pain but also the non-neurological causes. In one study in patients with PD, pain *related* to PD was as common as pain *unrelated* to PD (62.6 % vs. 64.2 %). Moreover, the pain in the latter group was rated by patients as significantly more severe and constant [71].

The pathogenesis of pain related to neurological conditions is complex. The basal ganglia have a crucial role in processing pain, and other somatosensory inputs and damage to these areas may affect how pain is perceived [72]. The basal ganglia can be affected in a number of neurodegenerative conditions (e.g., PD, PSP, MSA, HD, and stroke) and as such has been implicated as a mechanism for pain in these conditions.

As a whole, pain is common in neurodegenerative diseases:

- PD – Estimates of the frequency of pain in PD range from 40 to 85 % [71, 73]. It is more frequent when compared to an age-matched control group [74]. PD-related pains (such as cramps or dystonias) may worsen at "wearing off" times and improve with dopaminergic therapy. Other pains were thought to be non-PD related (mainly osteoarthritis). In all the studies, neuropathic pain was uncommon (<10 %).
- MS – The frequency of pain ranges from 29 to 86 % [75, 76]. The MS-related pains appear to be commonly due to neuropathic phenomenon but can also be related to spasticity.
- MND – Pain in MND tends to be more of an issue in later disease, and the prevalence has been estimated between 40 and 73 % [77]. It can be caused by cramps, spasticity, joint stiffness, or skin pressure due to immobility.

- Stroke – Pain post stroke has been shown to change with time. One population-based study demonstrated a prevalence of moderate/severe pain in 32 % of patients at 4 months and 21 % at 16 months [78]. They highlight the wide variations in estimates of pain post stroke (19–74 %) and that shoulder pain (on the affected side) and central post-stroke pain are most commonly reported.
- MSA/PSP – Pain in MSA has been reported in 47 % of patients in one retrospective study [79]. The pain was classified as "rheumatic," sensory, or dystonic with some evidence of exacerbation on "wearing off." Pain seems to affect patients with MSA much more commonly than patients with PSP (78 % vs. 56 %, respectively) [80].
- The prevalence of pain in HD is unknown, but one study found increased levels of bodily pain when compared to control norms [81]. The nature of the pain was not reported.

Management

The key element to optimal pain control is optimal pain assessment. All patients should have thorough assessments of each pain, and then treatments should be prescribed accordingly.

Nondrug

- Physiotherapy.
- Walking aids may help where pain is exacerbated by mobilization.
- Pressure-relieving devices (e.g., high-specification foam mattresses and cushions) to help treat or reduce risk of pressure sores.
- Transcutaneous electrical nerve stimulation (TENS) machine may be useful for some patients with chronic pain [82].
- Small benefits to chronic pain have also been demonstrated using psychological therapies [83].

Drug

Robust interventional studies looking at the drug treatments of pain in neurological conditions are lacking. However, evidence does suggest that analgesics are underused in patients with neurological conditions who have pain [71, 84].

In considering drug treatments, we will consider interventions under the proposed mechanism of the pain:

- Nociceptive pain:
  - In PD, optimizing dopaminergic therapy may help to alleviate pain in some patients.

- The WHO analgesic ladder [85] initially provided a useful structured approach to cancer pain management and may be useful in neurological conditions.

- Neuropathic pain:

  - Most RCTs for neuropathic pain have been undertaken in post-herpetic neuralgia and diabetic neuropathy. Evidence-based guidelines [86, 87] support the use of the following drugs for neuropathic pain. Use of any drug must weigh the risks and benefits associated:

  - Tricyclic antidepressants (e.g., amitriptyline)
  Other antidepressants (e.g., duloxetine)
  - Anticonvulsants (e.g., gabapentin, pregabalin)
  - Opioids (e.g., tramadol, morphine, oxycodone)
  - Topical lidocaine patches
  - Capsaicin patches

  - A review of pain in MS also suggests the use of carbamazepine or lamotrigine for painful paroxysms of pain (e.g., trigeminal neuralgia) [88].

Sleep Disorders

Neurodegenerative conditions can have a significant effect on sleep through a variety of mechanisms. Some of these may be:

1. Related directly to the neurological condition (e.g., REM sleep behavior disorder, obstructive sleep apnea syndrome, sleep hypoventilation syndrome, restless legs syndrome, or nocturnal akinesia) [89]
2. Indirectly related or even unrelated to the neurological condition (e.g., uncontrolled pain, symptoms, or depression)

A full assessment is therefore required to determine underlying causes of poor sleep and any reversible factors. Good "sleep hygiene" is still recommended for insomnia in non-neurological conditions, but robust evidence of its efficacy is not available [90]. For the purposes of this short section, however, we will focus on the more common sleep disorders which occur in neurodegenerative conditions.

REM Sleep Behavior Disorder (RBD)

This condition is characterized by vigorous movement and associated vivid and enacted unpleasant dreams during REM sleep. These movements can often cause injury to both patients and relatives. It is particularly common in multisystem atrophy (MSA), Parkinson's disease (PD), and diffuse Lewy body disease (LBD) with the prevalence ranging from 19 to 77 % [91]. Indeed, the occurrence of isolated RBD is significantly associated with the development of these neurodegenerative conditions with a 10-year risk of 40.6 % [92]. RBD has also been described in PSP and MS though less commonly. The diagnosis is confirmed by polysomnography which can also help to exclude other conditions.

Management

- There are no large controlled studies for the treatment of RBD; however, clonazepam is considered the treatment of choice on case series [93]. Second-line treatment with melatonin has been suggested [94].

Sleep Hypoventilation Syndrome

This syndrome is most commonly associated with motor neuron disease and is primarily related to the progressive weakness of the respiratory muscles. Symptomatic nocturnal hypoventilation leads to sleep fragmentation, daytime somnolence, poor concentration, and morning headaches. However, even prior to the development of symptoms, both bulbar weakness and mild diaphragmatic weakness can lead to objective sleep disturbance in early MND [95].

Management

- In order to alleviate the symptoms associated with respiratory dysfunction, the use of mechanical ventilation (tracheal ventilation [TV] or noninvasive ventilation [NIV]) in MND has becomes widespread. TV is more commonly used in Japan [96], while NIV is more commonly used worldwide. NIV can be delivered through a face or nasal mask and provides intermittent positive-pressure ventilation to patients with symptoms due to respiratory muscle weakness. An RCT by Bourke et al. [97] demonstrated that in those patients receiving NIV with normal or only moderately impaired bulbar function, there was improved symptom control, improved quality of life, and improved survival (median = 205 days). The National Institute for Health and Clinical Excellence (NICE) highlights the need for multidisciplinary team involvement and careful discussions with both patient and family when considering and using NIV [98].

Obstructive Sleep Apnea (OSA)

OSA is the occurrence of periods of reduced or pauses in breathing which are associated with narrowing or blockage of the airway during sleep. It is a condition which is associated with sleep fragmentation and daytime sleepiness.

In multiple system atrophy, patients can develop vocal cord dysfunction leading to laryngeal stridor and the development of OSA. Stridor is present in around 20 % of patients with MSA [99] and is associated with a poorer prognosis [100].

- *Treatment* with noninvasive positive-pressure ventilation (NIPPV) [101] and continuous positive airway pressure (CPAP) [102] in small case series have demonstrated an improvement in nocturnal stridor and hypoxemia during sleep. Longer-term follow-up in the use of CPAP also showed that the treatment was well tolerated, improved sleep quality, and may improve survival [103]. Excessive daytime sleepiness may well be a consequence of OSA in MSA, and a drug such as modafinil may have a role in symptomatic relief [104]. It may also have a role in PD [54].

Restless Legs Syndrome (RLS)

RLS is defined as an urge to move the legs which is usually accompanied by an uncomfortable or unpleasant sensation in the legs. It can begin or worsen during inactivity, be partially or totally relieved by movement, and is worse in the evening or at night [105]. It is prevalent in around 10 % of the population as a whole and tends to be more common in females [106]. RLS may be a significant and potentially treatable cause of sleep disturbance in patients with neurological conditions.

RLS is classified as primary or secondary. Primary RLS tends to be familial whereas secondary RLS is associated with other pathological conditions (such as neuropathies, uremia, and pregnancy).

- *Management* of RLS has largely focused on medications. As central dopaminergic systems have been implicated in the mechanisms of RLS, much of the treatment has focused on dopaminergic therapy:
  - Dopamine agonists (i.e., pramipexole, ropinirole, and rotigotine) have proven to be effective in systematic reviews. There is some evidence for their greater efficacy on RLS than levodopa [107].
  - Levodopa (100–200 mg at night) has also been shown to improve RLS, quality of life, and quality of sleep in short-term studies (1–8 weeks) [108]. Short-term use has been recommended because of the phenomenon of augmentation which has been described as a complication of levodopa in RLS. This resolves on discontinuation of treatment.
  - Other drugs which have shown efficacy and are recommended in RLS are opioids (e.g., oxycodone), anticonvulsants (e.g., gabapentin, carbamazepine, and valproate), and benzodiazepines (e.g., clonazepam) [109].

Spasticity

Spasticity is defined as a velocity-dependent increase in muscle tone and is associated with increased reflexes. It is a symptom which is common in neurodegenerative conditions (especially MS and stroke disease). Spasticity can adversely affect the ability to carry out daily tasks and is often described as stiffness or tightness in the affected area. It can lead to pain and also the development of contractures.

Management

Liaison with rehabilitation services can be helpful in complex cases.

Nondrug

- Spasticity can be exacerbated by many causes such as underlying infection, urinary retention, constipation, positional issues, or even ill-fitting footwear. Assessment for and treatment of underlying factors are important.
- Physiotherapy:
  - Stretching provides good immediate positive effects on spasticity; however, a systematic review of the evidence is inconclusive [110].
- Hydrotherapy or reflexology may also offer benefit [111].

Drug

- Anti-spasticity drugs – The most commonly used agents are baclofen, tizanidine, diazepam, and dantrolene. Two systematic reviews of their use in MS [112, 113] showed benefits in spasticity but failed to demonstrate any particular advantage of one drug over another and their use needs to be tailored to each patient:
  - Baclofen – It is an aminobutyric acid analogue and acts upon GABA receptors (gamma aminobutyric acid) mainly in the spinal cord by inhibiting glutamate release. It can cause drowsiness and muscle hypotonia.
  - Tizanidine – Acts principally at spinal cord level through presynaptic alpha-2 receptors. It also has central effects and can cause drowsiness and hypotension.
  - Diazepam – Acts at spinal and supraspinal levels via GABA receptors. It has a long plasma half-life and can cause drowsiness and muscle hypotonia.
  - Dantrolene – Acts directly on skeletal muscle and can cause muscle weakness. Liver function tests should be monitored regularly.
- Other drugs:
  - Cannabinoids – Acts on central cannabinoid receptors. In a large multicenter study, cannabinoids had little objective effect on spasticity but did appear to subjectively improve symptoms [114].

- – Levetiracetam [115], gabapentin [116], and pregabalin [117] have all shown promise, but further work is required.
- Botulinum toxin injections:
  - – There is excellent evidence for the efficacy and safety of the use of botulinum toxin in the treatment of spasticity [118].
- Intrathecal baclofen:
  - – Intrathecal baclofen has been used successfully for refractory spasticity in upper motor neuron lesions. Direct infusion into the intrathecal space allows higher drug levels at spinal level and with fewer systemic side effects. A review of its use showed both short- and long-term reduction in spasticity and suggested some functional and pain benefits [119].

Thickened Oral/Bronchial Secretions

Thick oral secretions have been recognized as a problem in the context of MND [77], but there is little published data in other neurodegenerative conditions. However, a number of treatment options are currently used clinically:

Management

Nondrug

- The use of oral hygiene, increased fluid intake, papaya enzymes, pineapple, chewing gum, saline nebulizers, or mucolytics have all been recommended. However, good evidence of their efficacy is lacking.
- Treat any underlying upper or lower respiratory tract infection. Exclude sinusitis and/or postnasal drip.

Drug

- Humidifiers, mucolytics, nebulizers (saline, beta-2 receptor agonists, anticholinergic bronchodilators), or furosemide have all been recommended, but there are no controlled trials [57].
- Studies in children have shown that thick secretions may be caused by the use of anticholinergic medication (e.g., glycopyrrolate [120]) or botulinum toxin [121], and therefore, dose reduction may be useful.
- While more thin serous secretions are largely under cholinergic control, the more thick mucoid secretions are under beta-adrenergic control. A small cases series suggested that beta-blockers, such as propanolol, can therefore help [122].

Physical

- In those patients with an ineffective cough due to respiratory muscle weakness, the use of mechanical insufflation/exsufflation or manually assisted cough can be helpful in clearing upper airway secretions [29]. This may be particularly helpful in acute infections. Physiotherapy may also have a role to play.
- Room humidification may help.
- Suction machines are commonly used to help clear thick tenacious secretions.

Urinary Symptoms

Urinary symptoms are another largely autonomically mediated complication of neurological conditions. However, there are very many secondary causes (e.g., poor mobility or drugs) which can themselves cause or compound urological problems.

In MS, bladder symptoms such as urgency, frequency, and urge incontinence occur in around 75 % of patients [123]. In urodynamic terms, these symptoms are caused by:

- Detrusor hyperreflexia (leading to urgency, frequency, and urge incontinence)
- Detrusor-sphincter dyssynergy where bladder contraction and sphincter release are uncoordinated – leading to hesitancy, interrupted stream, and incomplete emptying
- Detrusor hyporeflexia (residual urine, frequency)

Urodynamic assessment in patients with both MSA and PD demonstrated that patients with MSA had detrusor hyperreflexia in 81 % of cases whereas in PD it occurred in 56 %. Furthermore, detrusor-sphincter dyssynergy appeared to be more common in MSA [124]. A further study in PD showed detrusor hyporeflexia or areflexia in 16 % [125] leading to residual urine volumes. It is worth noting that these findings could occur in early disease.

Studies in stroke patients have demonstrated evidence of detrusor hyperactivity and underactivity in patients with dominant, nondominant, and bilateral hemispheric strokes [126, 127].

The evidence of autonomic involvement in MND may infer a primary mechanism for urinary symptoms; however, in reality, it is likely that the major contributing factors are the practicalities of micturition when the patient is immobile.

Management

Given the high prevalence of these symptoms in neurological conditions, any patient with urological symptoms requires a full assessment and individualized treatment.

Most of the studies looking at bladder symptoms in neurological conditions have occurred in MS, and from this limited evidence, the treatment recommendations below have been derived [12, 128]. Other guidance for long-term neurological conditions exists (e.g., PD [54]).

Investigations

- Exclude urinary tract infections or other underlying causes
- Post-micturition residual volumes using ultrasound scanning. This will help determine how efficiently the bladder is emptying.

Nondrug

- General measures for treating incontinence or urgency such as avoiding coffee/alcohol or limiting water intake (1–1.5 l).
- Review current medication (e.g., diuretics)
- Advice on toileting arrangements or clothing to help access in cases of urge incontinence
- Behavioral techniques such as pelvic floor exercises or neuromuscular stimulation (electrical stimulation to pudendal nerve to help pelvic floor contractions) [129] have shown positive effects when used together in some MS patients.

Drug

- For urge incontinence or urgency, where conservative measures have failed, anticholinergics (e.g., oxybutynin and tolterodine) have proven to be effective in systematic reviews in non-neurological conditions [130, 131]. Any use should be regularly reviewed as they can precipitate urinary retention, dry mouth, and other side effects such as confusion. In general, side effects are better with tolterodine immediate release versus oxybutynin IR, while controlled release (CR) preparations are better tolerated than IR.
  - In this systematic review, the newer anticholinergic solifenacin appeared to be more efficacious and less likely to cause dry mouth.
  - Intravesical atropine [132] and transdermal oxybutynin [133] have also been used for detrusor overactivity and may be associated with fewer anticholinergic side effects.
- Desmopressin (a synthetic vasopressin analogue) which has been recommended as a short-term (<6 h) measure to control frequency.
  - A metanalysis in desmopressin use in MS demonstrated a moderate improvement in frequency [134]. Rarely, serum sodium can drop and should therefore be monitored.
  - Desmopressin may be useful in other neurological conditions (PD [135] MSA [136]).

- Botulinum toxin A injection into overactive detrusor muscle has shown promising results in systematic reviews [137]. Longer-term studies in MS have demonstrated an improvement in quality of life and a median time to retreatment of 12–13 months [138].
  - A small case series in PD and MSA also showed some benefit in urinary frequency and increased quality of life [139].
- In PD, optimizing dopaminergic therapy may have a role.

Use of catheterization for refractory cases

- If there is a high residual volume in the bladder and the patient is able consider intermittent self-catheterization (ISC). These are most commonly used in MS or spinal cord dysfunction, and their use is associated with fewer infections and decreased bacteriuria when compared to indwelling catheters [140]. The use of ISC in other conditions is often limited by the accompanying physical disabilities and practicalities of self-insertion.
- Guidelines in MS regarding long-term indwelling catheters suggest that they should only be used when all reasonable noninvasive methods have been tried and that once in use, they should be reviewed regularly [12]. The use of indwelling catheters in general have been recommended in other circumstances such as:
  - Chronic urinary retention
  - Skins which are being contaminated by urine
  - Distress caused by bed and clothing changes [141]
- Suprapubic catheters are recommended in long-term use in order to reduce the risk of urethral damage in MS patients [128]. Though they are not without complications, overall satisfaction with suprapubic catheters is high [142].

Treatment for Symptoms Which Are Specific to Particular Neurological Conditions

In this section, we will briefly look at some disease-specific symptoms and their management.

Parkinson's Disease

Parkinson's disease patients have a particular cluster of symptoms which can be challenging to manage especially in advanced disease. Liaison with or referral to local specialist PD services is recommended in more complex cases.

Rigidity and Dystonia

Muscle stiffness in the context of parkinsonian disorders (i.e., PD/ MSA/ PSP) can be due to rigidity or dystonia.

- *Rigidity* is present throughout passive movement and is not velocity dependent (unlike spasticity). If symptomatic for the patient, it may respond to reviewing dopaminergic treatment.
- *Dystonia* is an involuntary muscle contraction which can force the body into abnormal and sometimes painful postures. In the context of PD, this commonly occurs in the feet, tend to occur in the "off" phase, and can respond to:

  - Altering the dopaminergic regime to reduce "off" phases
  - Botulinum toxin injection to the affected area
  - Deep brain stimulation [143]

Dyskinesia

Dyskinesia is a general term which describes family of involuntary movements in a number of conditions. In PD, dyskinesia most commonly associated with the use of levodopa though other mechanisms are postulated. Estimates of its prevalence vary, but one review found that nearly 40 % of patients had dyskinesia after 4–6 years of levodopa treatment [144]. It tends to be more common in those whose PD started at a younger age [145]. Dyskinesias can be very disabling and are associated with a poorer quality of life [146].

The commonest form of dyskinesia in PD is peak-dose dyskinesia which can involve any part of the body (commonly the limbs, but it can affect swallowing and respiratory function). Biphasic dyskinesias (or diphasic) are less common and occur at the onset and end of dose. They tend to affect the lower limbs more and are associated with more pain [147]. Both peak-dose and biphasic dyskinesias can occur in the same patient.

Levodopa-induced dyskinesia has been reported in MSA and PSP but to a lesser extent than in PD. This finding may in part reflect the lower use of levodopa in these groups as well as a poorer response rate to the drug [148].

Management

Nondrug
- Use of daily diaries can help to clarify the pattern of the dyskinesia and its relationship to drug administration.

Drug
- Optimize dopaminergic regime

  - Reduce the individual doses of dopamine but increase the number of daily doses.

- *Otherwise* consider reducing dose of drugs such as monoamine oxidase B inhibitors (e.g., selegiline) or catechol-O-methyltransferase inhibitors (COMT) such as entacapone.
- Advice for other changes should be sought from specialist PD teams (especially in biphasic dyskinesias).

• Amantadine (200–400 mg/day) has been recommended for use in dyskinesias though systematic reviews suggest a lack of evidence for its efficacy [149].

Surgical

• Deep brain stimulation of the subthalamic nucleus has been shown to be effective in refractory cases [150].

Hallucinations

A review of hallucinations in PD demonstrated that between 8 and 40 % of patients on long-term treatment have visual hallucinations during their illness [151]. The cause of hallucinations is complex and can be related to:

• The parkinsonian disorder itself:

- This tends to be found in late-stage PD and is associated with the development of cortical Lewy bodies.
- The development of hallucinations *early* in the course of a parkinsonian disorder raises the question of dementia with Lewy bodies (DLB). Other features such as cognitive decline, pronounced cognitive fluctuations, and parkinsonism should be assessed [152]. Furthermore, 50 % of patients with DLB show neuroleptic sensitivity reactions [153] and as such these drugs should be used cautiously.

• Secondary issues including:

- Background issues – age, cognitive impairment, comorbid conditions
- Medications – antiparkinsonian or other drugs (e.g., anticholinergics/ sedatives)
- Infection

Management

• Full history and examination with appropriate investigations.
• Reverse any underlying cause.

- Full explanation to patient and family:
    - If hallucinations are not troublesome, consider watch and wait policy after discussion with patient and family
- Consider staggered withdrawal of the antiparkinsonian medication:
    - Recommended order of withdrawal (first to last) of anticholinergics, amantadine, MAOI-B inhibitors, COMT inhibitors, and then lastly levodopa [143].
    - Any withdrawal needs to be balanced with the potential worsening of motor symptoms.
- Atypical antipsychotic such as quetiapine and clozapine [154] has been shown to be effective. However, there is a risk of agranulocytosis with clozapine, so blood tests should be monitored. (NB – typical antipsychotics should be avoided).
- Cholinesterase inhibitors (e.g., rivastigmine) have also been efficacious in small studies [155].

Nausea and Vomiting

We mention nausea and vomiting in PD not because it is a particularly common symptom (~10 % [1]) but rather because of the challenges it raises in treatment. Many of the drugs used to treat nausea and vomiting have actions on the central dopaminergic pathways and, as such, can cause worsening of parkinsonian symptoms (in PD, PSP, and MSA). These drugs include haloperidol, metoclopramide, prochlorperazine, levomepromazine, and cyclizine.

Management

Nondrug

- The role of acupuncture for sickness has yet to be elucidated, but it has shown efficacy in systematic reviews of chemotherapy-induced vomiting [156].

Drugs

- Domperidone does not cross the blood-brain barrier and as such can be used for nausea and vomiting related to gastric stasis [143].
- Ondansetron does not worsen parkinsonism [157] and therefore can be safely used for nausea mediated through the chemoreceptor trigger zone. Bowel habit needs to be closely monitored as it can cause constipation.
- Hyoscine hydrobromide has been used as a treatment for PD [158] prior to the widespread use of levodopa. It can be administered orally, transdermally (as a patch), or by injection. Its use as an antiemetic in PD, however, may be limited in view of its anticholinergic side effects (e.g., drowsiness and confusion).

Progressive Supranuclear Palsy

Visual Problems

One of the distinguishing features of PSP from other parkinsonian diseases is the development of eye signs. One study [14] of 187 PSP patients demonstrated the frequency of the signs:

- Vertical gaze palsy = 94 %
- Diplopia/blurred vision = 39 %
- Photophobia = 20 %
- Eyelid apraxia (inability to voluntarily open the eyes) = 17 %

Interestingly patients were more likely to complain of the symptoms of diplopia/ blurred vision, photophobia, and eyelid apraxia. Blepharospasm (a repetitive involuntary sustained contraction of the orbicularis oculi muscle which closes the eye) is a focal dystonia which has also been described in PSP [159].

Management

There are few published studies looking at the treatment of eye problems in PSP.
- Patients with photophobia may benefit from sunglasses which may need to be worn indoors and outdoors.
- Eyelid apraxia and blepharospasm

  - Various physical means have been tried to help keep the eyes open in eyelid apraxia [160].
  - Local botulinum toxin injections have proved beneficial for both eyelid apraxia and blepharospasm [161, 162].

- Diplopia or difficulty with downward gaze may need referral for an ophthalmology assessment.

  - Prisms may have a role in alleviating symptoms and improving ability to carry out daily activities [163].

Multiple Sclerosis

Ataxia

Ataxia is the loss of muscular coordination and is present in up to 80 % of patients with MS at some point in their disease course [164]. It appears, in part, to be associated with MRI changes in the infratentorial area [165]. These infratentorial lesions in turn are associated with an increased risk of problems with standing balance and with falls [166].

Management

- A systematic review of non-pharmacological, pharmacological, and surgical interventions in MS patients with ataxia demonstrated only short-term benefit from some therapies (physiotherapy, neurorehabilitation, and surgery) [167].
- Recommendations for treatment of ataxia in MS therefore involve referral to specialist neurorehabilitation teams and, in severe refractory cases, consideration of neurosurgery [12].

Huntington's Disease

Chorea

Chorea is defined as involuntary, purposeless, jerking, or twitching movements. In HD, the chorea is a feature (31–36 %) of early disease (<5 years) which then tends to become less common as the disease progresses (6–13 % in >6 years) [168]. These abnormal movements are thought to be mediated through central dopaminergic and glutamatergic systems, and as such, these neurotransmitter systems have been the focus of drug therapies [169].

Management

Liaison with local Huntington's disease services is recommended.

Drug

- Antidopaminergic

  - Tetrabenazine (up to 100 mg/day) depletes presynaptic dopamine in the central nervous system and has been found to decrease chorea in patients with HD [170]. The side effects include drowsiness and depression.
  - Sulpiride (900–1,200 mg/day) is another antidopaminergic drug which has been shown to be effective for chorea in a small trial. Again, the most common side effect was drowsiness in HD, though parkinsonism and akathisia were described with its use in other conditions [171].

- Antiglutamatergic

  - Amantadine and riluzole had mixed results when assessed in a systematic review [172].

Conclusion

This chapter has considered the physical aspects of symptom control in multiple sclerosis (MS), Parkinson's disease (PD), progressive supranuclear palsy (PSP), multiple system atrophy (MSA), motor neuron disease (MND), Huntington's disease (HD), and stroke disease. As highlighted in the case study and throughout the chapter, these symptoms are optimally treated through a combination of careful patient-centered assessment, timely intervention, open and honest discussion, realistic goal setting, planning ahead, coordination of care, and regular review of patient and carer.

References

1. Lee MA, Prentice WM, Hildreth AJ, Walker RW. Measuring symptom load in idiopathic Parkinson's disease. Parkinsonism Relat Disord. 2007;13(5):284–9.
2. Visser M, Marinus J, van Hilton JJ, Schipper RGB, Stiggelbout M. Assessing comorbidity in patients with Parkinson's disease. Mov Disord. 2004;19(7):824–8.
3. Marrie RA, Horwitz RI. Emerging effects of comorbidities on multiple sclerosis. Lancet Neurol. 2010;9(8):820–8.
4. Papapetropoulos S, Singer C, McCorquodale D, Gonzalez J, Mash DC. Cause, seasonality of death and co-morbidities in progressive supranuclear palsy. Parkinsonism Relat Disord. 2005;11(7):459–63.
5. Parkinson's Disease Society of the UK. Life with PD today – room for improvement. London: Parkinson's Disease Society; 2008.
6. Bromberg MB, Forshew DA. Comparison of instruments addressing quality of life in patients with ALS and their caregivers. Neurology. 2002;58:320–2.
7. The National Council of Palliative Care. Addressing the palliative care for people with neurological conditions. Focus on neurology. London: The National Council of Palliative Care; 2007.
8. National End of Life Care Programme/National Council for Palliative Care/The Neurological Alliance. Improving end of life care in neurological disease a framework for implementation. 2010. http://www.endoflifecareforadults.nhs.uk/publications/end-of-life-care-in-long-term-neurological-conditions-a-framework. Accessed 15 Apr 2012.
9. The National Council of Palliative Care. Exploring the interface: a survey of neurology nurses' involvement with Specialist Palliative Care Services and identification of their training needs. London: The National Council of Palliative Care and The Royal College of Nursing; 2008.
10. O'Brien T, Kelly M, Saunders C. Motor neurone disease: a hospice perspective. BMJ. 1992;304:471–3.
11. Hicks F, Corcoran G. Should hospices offer respite admissions to patients with motor neurone disease? Palliat Med. 1993;7:145–50.
12. National Collaborating Centre for Chronic Conditions. Multiple sclerosis: national clinical guidelines for diagnosis and management in primary and secondary care. London: Royal College of Physicians; 2004.
13. Bulpitt CJ, Shaw K, Clifton P, Stern G, Davies JB, Reid JL. The symptoms of patients treated for Parkinson's disease. Clin Neuropharmacol. 1985;8(2):175–83.
14. Nath U, Ben-Schlomo Y, Thomson RG, Lees AJ, Burn DJ. Clinical features and natural history of progressive supranuclear palsy: a clinical cohort study. Neurology. 2003;60(6):910–6.

15. Sjostrom AC, Holmberg B, Strang P. Parkinson-plus patients – an unknown group with severe symptoms. J Neurosci Nurs. 2002;34(6):314–9.
16. World Health Organisation. National cancer control programmes: policies and managerial guidelines. 2nd ed. Geneva: World Health Organisation; 2002.
17. Department of Health. The national service framework for long-term (neurological) conditions. London: HMSO; 2005.
18. Miller RG, Mitchell JD, Moore DH. Riluzole for amyotrophic lateral sclerosis(ALS)/motor neuron disease (MND). Cochrane Database Syst Rev. 2012;3:CD001447.
19. Orrell RW, Lane RJM, Ross M. Antioxidant treatment for amyotrophic lateral sclerosis or motor neuron disease. Cochrane Database Syst Rev. 2007;1:CD002829.
20. Carter L. The management of medication for Parkinson's disease in hospital and care homes. Br J Neurosci Nurs. 2006;2(6):281–5.
21. Adler CH. Nonmotor complications in Parkinson's disease. Mov Disord. 2005;20(11):S23–9.
22. Stacy M. The wearing-off phenomenon and the use of questionnaires to facilitate its recognition in Parkinson's disease. J Neural Transm. 2010;117:837–46.
23. Stacy MA, Murck H, Kroenke K. Responsiveness of motor and nonmotor symptoms of Parkinson's disease to dopaminergic therapy. Prog Neuropsychopharmacol Biol Psychiatry. 2010;34:57–61.
24. Sellebjerg F, Barnes D, Filippini G, et al. EFNS guideline on treatment of multiple sclerosis relapses: report of an EFNS task force on treatment of multiple sclerosis relapses. Eur J Neurol. 2006;12:939–46.
25. Mehanna R, Jankovic J. Respiratory problems in neurologic movement disorders. Parkinsonism Relat Disord. 2010;16(10):628–38.
26. Mutluay FK, Gurses HN, Saip H. Effects of multiple sclerosis on respiratory function. Clin Rehabil. 2005;19(4):426–32.
27. American Thoracic Society. Dyspnea. Mechanisms, assessment, and management: a consensus statement. Am J Respir Crit Care Med. 1999;159:321–40.
28. Weiner P, Inzelberg R, Davidovich A, et al. Respiratory muscle performance and the perception of dyspnea in Parkinson's disease. Can J Neurol Sci. 2002;29(1):68–72.
29. Miller RG, Jackson CE, Karsarskis EJ, et al. Practice parameters: the care of the patient with amyotrophic lateral sclerosis: drug, nutritional, and respiratory therapies (an evidence-based review). Report of the quality standards subcommittee of the American Academy of Neurology. Neurology. 2009;73:1218–26.
30. Bausewein C, Booth S, Gysels M, et al. Non-pharmacological interventions for breathlessness in advanced stages of malignancy and non-malignant disease. Cochrane Database Syst Rev. 2008;2:CD005623.
31. Jennings AL, Davies AN, Higgins JPT, et al. Opioids for the palliation of breathlessness in advanced disease and terminal illness. Cochrane Database Syst Rev. 2001;3:CD002066.
32. Simon ST, Higginson IJ, Booth S, et al. Benzodiazepines for the relief of breathlessness in advanced malignant and non-malignant diseases. Cochrane Database Syst Rev. 2010;1: CD007354.
33. Longstreth GF, Thompson WG, Chey WD, Houghton LA, Mearin F, Spiller RC. Functional bowel disorders. Gastroenterology. 2006;130(5):1480–91.
34. Lee-Robichaud H, Thomas K, Morgan J, Nelson RL. Lactulose versus Polyethylene Glycol for chronic constipation. Cochrane Database Syst Rev. 2010;7:CD007570.
35. Muller-Lissner S, Rykx A, Kerstens R, Vandeplassche L. A double blind, placebo controlled study of prucalopride in elderly patients with constipation. Neurogastroenterol Motil. 2010; 22(9):991–8.
36. Liu Z, Sakakibara R, Odaka T, et al. Mosapride citrate, a novel 5HT4 agonist and partial 5HT3 antagonist, ameliorates constipation in parkinsonian patients. Mov Disord. 2005;20(6): 680–6.
37. Bradley WG, Anderson F, Bromberg M, et al. Current management of ALS: comparison of the ALS CARE database and the ANN practice parameter. Neurology. 2001;57(3):500–4.

38. Kalf JG, de Swart BJ, Borm GF, Bloem BR, Munneke M. Prevalence and definition of drooling in Parkinson's disease: a systematic review. J Neurol. 2009;256(9):1391–6.
39. Charchaflie RJ, Bustos-Fernandez L, Perec CJ, Gonzalez E, Marzi A. Functional studies of the parotid and pancreas glands in amyotrophic lateral sclerosis. J Neurol Neurosurg Psychiatry. 1974;37(7):863–7.
40. Nobrega AC, Rodrigues B, Torres AC, Scarpel RD, Neves CA, Melo A. Is drooling secondary to a swallowing disorder in patients with Parkinson's disease? Parkinsonism Relat Disord. 2008;14(3):243–5.
41. Pehlivan M, Yuceyar N, Ertekin C, et al. An electronic device measuring the frequency of spontaneous swallowing: digital phagometer. Dysphagia. 1996;11(4):259–64.
42. Marks L, Turner K, O'Sullivan J, Deighton B, Lees A. Drooling in Parkinson's disease: a novel speech and language therapy intervention. Int J Lang Commun Disord. 2001;36(Suppl): 282–7.
43. South AR, Summers SM, Jog MS. Gum chewing improves swallow frequency and latency in Parkinson's patients. A preliminary study. J Neurol. 2010;74(15):1198–202.
44. Jongerius PH, van Tiel P, van Limbeek J, Gabreels FJM, Rotteveel JJ. A systematic review for evidence of efficacy of anticholinergic drugs to treat drooling. Arch Dis Child. 2003;88(10): 911–4.
45. De Simone GG, Eisenchlas JH, Junin M, Pereyra F, Brizuela R. Atropine drops for drooling: a randomised control trial. Palliat Med. 2006;20(7):665–71.
46. Mato A, Jacobo L, Inmaculada T, Munoz M, Concepcion A. Management of drooling in disabled patients with scopolamine patches. Br J Clin Pharmacol. 2010;69(6):684–8.
47. Arbouw MEL, Movig KLL, Koopman M, et al. Glycopyrrolate for sialorrhea in PD: a randomised, double blind, crossover trial. Neurology. 2010;74(15):1203–7.
48. Reddihough D, Erasmus CE, Johnson H, McKellar GMW, Jongerius PH. Botulinum toxin assessment, intervention and aftercare for paediatric and adult drooling: international consensus statement. Eur J Neurol. 2010;17 Suppl 2:109–21.
49. Neppelberg E, Haugen DF, Thorsen L, Tysnes OB. Radiotherapy reduces sialorrhea in amyotrophic lateral sclerosis. Eur J Neurol. 2007;14(12):1373–7.
50. Voltz R, Borasio GD. Palliative therapy in the terminal stage of neurological disease. J Neurol. 1997;244 Suppl 4:s2–10.
51. Miller N, Allcock L, Jones D, Noble E, Hildreth AJ, Burn DJ. Prevalence and pattern of perceived intelligibilty changes in Parkinson's disease. J Neurol Neurosurg Psychiatry. 2007;78:1 188–90.
52. Ramig LO, Sapir S, Fox C, Countryman S. Changes in vocal loudness following intensive voice treatment (LSVT) in individuals with Parkinson's disease: a comparison with untreated patients and normal age-matched controls. Mov Disord. 2001;16(1):79–83.
53. Ertekin C, Aydogdu I. Neurophysiology of swallowing. Clin Neurophysiol. 2003;114(12): 2226–44.
54. National Collaborating Centre for Chronic Conditions. Parkinson's Disease: national clinical guidelines for diagnosis and management in primary and secondary care. London: Royal College of Physicians; 2006.
55. Hunter PC, Crameri J, Austin S, Woodward MC, Hughes AJ. Response of parkinsonian swallowing dysfunction to dopaminergic stimulation. J Neurol Neurosurg Psychiatry. 1997;63(5): 579–83.
56. Gomes Jr CAR, Lustosa SAS, Matos D, Andriolo RB, Waisberg DR, Waisberg J. Percutaneous endoscopic gastrostomy versus nasogastric tube feeding for adults with swallowing disturbances. Cochrane Database Syst Rev. 2010;11:CD008096.
57. Andersen PM, Borasio GD, Dengler R, et al. EFNS task force on the management of amyotrophic lateral sclerosis: guidelines for diagnosing and clinical care of patients and relatives. An evidence-based review with good practice points. Eur J Neurol. 2005;12: 921–38.
58. Antonini A, Mancini F, Canesi M, et al. Duodenal levodopa infusion improves quality of life in advanced Parkinson's disease. Neurodegener Dis. 2008;5(3–4):244–6.

59. Chaudhuri A, Behan BO. Fatigue in neurological disorders. Lancet. 2004;363(9413):978–88.
60. Kos D, Kerckhof E, Nagels G, D'hooghe MB, Ilsbroukx S. Origin of fatigue in multiple sclerosis: review of the literature. Neurorehabil Neural Repair. 2008;22(1):91–100.
61. Grossman P, Kappos L, Gensicke H, et al. MS quality of life, depression, and fatigue improve after mindfulness training: a randomized trial. Neurology. 2010;75(13):1141–9.
62. Tyne H, Taylor J, Baker GA, Steiger M. Modafinil for Parkinson's disease fatigue. J Neurol. 2010;257(3):452–6.
63. Rammohan KW, Rosenberg JH, Lynn DJ, Blumfeld AM, Pollak CP, Nagaraja HN. Efficacy and safety of modafinil (Provigil) for the treatment of fatigue in multiple sclerosis: a two centre phase 2 study. J Neurol Neurosurg Psychiatry. 2002;72(2):179–83.
64. Barnes MP. Principles of neurological rehabilitation. J Neurol Neurosurg Psychiatry. 2003;74(Suppl IV):3–7.
65. Busse ME, Khalil H, Quinn L, Rosser AE. Physical therapy intervention for people with Huntington's disease. Phys Ther. 2008;88(7):820–31.
66. Factor SA. The clinical spectrum of freezing gait in atypical parkinsonism. Mov Disord. 2008;23:S431–8.
67. Nieuwboer A. Cueing for freezing of gait inpatients with Parkinson's disease. Mov Disord. 2008;23:S475–81.
68. Gagliese L, Melzack R. Chronic pain in elderly people. Pain. 1997;70:3–14.
69. Elliott AM, Smith BH, Penny KI, Smith WC, Chambers WA. The epidemiology of chronic pain in the community. Lancet. 1999;354:1248–52.
70. Roy R, Thomas MR. Elderly persons with and without pain: a comparative study. Clin J Pain. 1987;3:102–6.
71. Lee MA, Walker RW, Hildreth TJ, Prentice WM. A survey of pain in idiopathic Parkinson's disease. J Pain Symptom Manage. 2006;32(5):462–9.
72. Chudler EH, Dong WK. The role of basal ganglia in nociception and pain. Pain. 1995; 60:3–38.
73. Ford B. Pain in Parkinson's disease. Clin Neurosci. 1998;5:63–72.
74. Defazio G, Berardelli A, Fabbrini G, et al. Pain as a non motor symptom of Parkinson disease. Evidence from a case–control study. Arch Neurol. 2008;65(9):1191–4.
75. Solaro C, Brichetto G, Amato MP, et al. The prevalence of pain in multiple sclerosis. A multicenter cross-sectional study. Neurology. 2004;63:919–21.
76. Brochet MB, Deloire MSA, Ouallet JC, et al. Pain and quality of life in the early stages after multiple sclerosis diagnosis: a 2-year longitudinal study. Clin J Pain. 2009;25(3):211–9.
77. Miller RG, Rosenberg JA, Gelinas DF, et al. Practice parameters: the care of the patient with amyotrophic lateral sclerosis (an evidence based review). Report of the quality standards subcommittee of the American Academy of Neurology. Neurology. 1999;52(7):1311–23.
78. Jonsson AC, Lindgren I, Hallstrom B, Norrving B, Lindgren A. Prevalence and intensity of pain after stroke: a population based study focusing on patients' perspectives. J Neurol Neurosurg Psychiatry. 2006;77(5):590–5.
79. Tison F, Wenning GK, Volonte MA, Poewe WR, Henry P, Quinn NP. Pain in multiple system atrophy. J Neurol. 1996;243(2):153–6.
80. Schrag A, Sheikh S, Quinn NP, et al. A comparison of depression, anxiety, and health status in patients with progressive supranuclear palsy and multiple system atrophy. Mov Disord. 2010;25(8):1077–81.
81. Ho AK, Gilbert AS, Mason SL, Goodman AO, Barker RA. Health-related quality of life in Huntington's disease: what factors matter most? Mov Disord. 2009;24(4):574–8.
82. Nnoaham KE, Kumbang J. Transcutaneous electrical nerve stimulation (TENS) for chronic pain. Cochrane Database Syst Rev. 2008;3:CD003222.
83. Eccleston C, Williams ACDC, Morley S. Psychological therapies for the management of chronic pain (excluding headaches) in adults. Cochrane Database Syst Rev. 2009;2: CD007407.
84. Solaro C, Brichetto G, Amato MP, et al. The prevalence of pain in multiple sclerosis. A multicenter cross-sectional study. Neurology. 2004;63:919–21.

85. World Health Organisation. Cancer pain relief. 2nd ed. Geneva: WHO; 1996.
86. NICE clinical guideline 96. Neuropathic pain: the pharmacological management of neuro-pathic pain in adults in non specialist settings. London: National Institute for Health and Clinical Excellence; 2010.
87. Dworkin RH, O'Connor AB, Backonja M, et al. Pharmacological management of neuro-pathic pain: evidence-based recommendations. Pain. 2007;132(3):237–51.
88. Pollman W, Feneberg W. Current management of pain associated with multiple sclerosis. CNS Drugs. 2008;22(4):291–324.
89. Jennum P, Santamaria Cano J, Basetti C, et al. Sleep disorders in neurodegenerative condi-tions and stroke disease. In: Gilhus NE, Barnes MP, Brainin M, editors. European handbook of neurological management. 2nd ed. West Sussex: Blackwell Publishing Ltd; 2011. p. 529–43.
90. Stepanski EJ, Wyatt JK. Use of sleep hygiene in the treatment of insomnia. Sleep Med Rev. 2003;7(3):215–25.
91. Thomas A, Bonanni L, Onofrj M. Symptomatic REM sleep behaviour disorder. Neurol Sci. 2007;28:S21–36.
92. Postuma RB, Gagnon JF, Vendette M, Fantini ML, Massicotte-Marquez J, Montplaisir J. Quantifying the risk of neurodegenerative disease in idiopathic REM sleep behavior disorder. Neurology. 2009;72(15):1296–300.
93. Lapierre O, Montplaisir J. Polysomnographic features of REM sleep behaviour disorder. Development of a scoring method. Neurology. 1992;42(7):1371–4.
94. Kunz D, Mahlberg R. A two part, double blind, placebo controlled trial of exogenous mela-tonin in REM sleep behaviour disorder. J Sleep Res. 2010;19(4):591–6.
95. Kimura K, Tachibana N, Kimura J, Shibasaki H. Sleep-disordered breathing at an early stage of amyotrophic lateral sclerosis. J Neurol Sci. 1999;164(1):37–43.
96. Hayashi H. Ventilatory support: Japanese experience. J Neurol Sci. 1997;152 Suppl 1: S97–100.
97. Bourke SC, Tomlinson M, Williams TL, Bullock RE, Shaw PJ, Gibson GJ. Effects of non-invasive ventilation on survival and quality of life in patients with amyotrophic lateral sclero-sis: a randomised controlled trial. Lancet Neurol. 2006;5(2):140–7.
98. National Institute for Health and Clinical Excellence. Motor Neurone Disease: the use of non-invasive ventilation in the management of motor neurone disease. NICE clinical guide-line 105. 2010. www.nice.org.uk/nicemedia/live/13057/49885/49885.pdf. Accessed 15 July 2011.
99. Plazzi G, Corsini R, Provini F, et al. REM sleep behaviour disorders in multiple system atro-phy. Neurology. 1997;48(4):1094–6.
100. Silber MH, Levine S. Stridor and death in multiple system atrophy. Mov Disord. 2000; 15(4):699–704.
101. Nonaka M, Imai T, Shintani T, Kawamata M, Chiba S, Matsumoto H. Non-invasive positive pressure ventilation for laryngeal contraction disorder during sleep in multiple system atro-phy. J Neurol Sci. 2006;247(1):53–8.
102. Iranzo A, Santamaria J, Tolosa E. Continuous positive air pressure eliminates nocturnal stri-dor in multiple system atrophy. Barcelona Multiple System Atrophy Study Group. Lancet. 2000;356(9238):1329–30.
103. Iranzo A, Santamaria J, Tolosa E, et al. Long term effect of CPAP in the treatment of noctur-nal stridor in multiple system atrophy. Neurology. 2004;63(5):930–2.
104. Arnulf I. Excess daytime sleepiness in parkinsonism. Sleep Med Rev. 2005;9(3):185–200.
105. Allen RP, Picchietti D, Hening WA, et al. Restless leg syndrome: diagnostic criteria, special considerations, and epidemiology. A report from the restless legs syndrome diagnosis and epidemiology workshop at the National Institutes of Health. Sleep Med. 2003;4(2): 101–19.
106. Berger K, Luedemann J, Trenkwalder C, John U, Kessler C. Sex and the risk of restless leg syndrome in the general population. Arch Intern Med. 2004;164(2):196–202.

107. Scholz H, Trenkwalder C, Kohnen R, Riemann D, Kriston L, Hornyak M. Dopamine agonists for the treatment of restless legs syndrome. Cochrane Database Syst Rev. 2011;3: CD006009.
108. Scholz H, Trenkwalder C, Kohnen R, Riemann D, Kriston L, Hornyak M. Levodopa for the treatment of restless legs syndrome. Cochrane Database Syst Rev. 2011;2:CD005504.
109. Vignatelli L, Billiard M, Clarenbach P, et al. EFNS guidelines on management of restless legs syndrome and periodic limb movement disorder in sleep. Eur J Neurol. 2006;13:1049–65.
110. Bovend'Eerdt TJ, Newman M, Barker K, Dawes H, Minelli C, Wade DT. The effects of stretching in spasticity: a systematic review. Arch Phys Med Rehabil. 2008;89(7):1395–406.
111. Pappalardo A, Castiglione A, Restivo DA, et al. Non-pharmacological interventions for spasticity associated with multiple sclerosis. Neurol Sci. 2006;27 Suppl 4:s316–9.
112. Shakespeare D, Boggild M, Young CA. Anti-spasticity agents for multiple sclerosis. Cochrane Database Syst Rev. 2003;4:CD001332.
113. Beard S, Hunn A, Wight J. Treatments for spasticity and pain in multiple sclerosis: a systematic review. Health Technol Assess. 2003;7(40):1–111.
114. Zajicek J, Fox P, Sanders H, et al. Cannabinoids for treatment of spasticity and other symptoms related to multiple sclerosis (CAMS study): multicentre randomised placebo-controlled trial. Lancet. 2003;362(9395):1517–26.
115. Bedlack RS, Pastula DM, Hawes J, Heydt D. Open-label pilot trial of levetiracetam for cramps and spasticity in patients with motor neuron disease. Amyotroph Lateral Scler. 2009;10(4):210–5.
116. Cutter NC, Scott DD, Johnson JC, Whiteneck G. Gabapentin effect on spasticity in multiple sclerosis: a placebo-controlled randomized trial. Arch Phys Med Rehabil. 2000;81(2): 164–9.
117. Bradley LJ, Kirker SGB. Pregabalin in the treatment of spasticity: a retrospective case series. Disabil Rehabil. 2008;30(16):1230–2.
118. Simpson DM, Gracies J-M, Graham HK, et al. Assessment: botulinum neurotoxin for the treatment of spasticity (an evidence-based review): report to the therapeutics and technology assessment subcommittee of the American Academy of Neurology. Neurology. 2008;70: 1691–8.
119. Rietman JS, Geertzen JHB. Efficacy of intrathecal baclofen delivery in the management of severe spasticity in upper motor neuron syndrome. Acta Neurochir Suppl. 2007;97(3): 205–11.
120. Bachrach SJ, Walter RS, Trzcinski K. Use of glycopyrrolate and other anticholinergic medications for sialorrhea in children with cerebral palsy. Clin Pediatr. 1998;37(8):485–90.
121. Erasmus CE, van Hulst K, van den Hoogen FJA, et al. Thickened saliva after effective management of drooling with botulinum toxin a. Dev Med Child Neurol. 2010;52(6):e114–8.
122. Newall AR, Orser R, Hunt M. The control of oral secretions in bulbar ALS/MND. J Neurol Sci. 1996;139 Suppl 1:43–4.
123. DasGupta R, Fowler CJ. Bladder, bowel and sexual dysfunction in multiple sclerosis: management strategies. Drugs. 2003;63(2):153–66.
124. Sakakibara R, Hattori T, Uchiyama T, Yamanishi T. Videodynamic and sphincter motor unit potential analyses in Parkinson's disease and multiple system atrophy. J Neurol Neurosurg Psychiatry. 2001;71(5):600–6.
125. Araki I, Kitahara M, Oida T, Kuno S. Voiding dysfunction and Parkinson's disease: urodynamic abnormalities and urinary symptoms. J Urol. 2000;164(5):1640–3.
126. Kim TG, Yoo KH, Jeon SH, Lee HL, Chang SG. Effect of dominant hemispheric stroke on detrusor function in patients with lower urinary tract symptoms. Int J Urol. 2010;17(7): 656–60.
127. Ersoz M, Tunc H, Akyuz M, Ozel S. Bladder storage and emptying disorder frequencies in hemorrhagic and ischemic stroke patients with bladder dysfunction. Cerebrovasc Dis. 2005;20(5):395–9.

128. Fowler CJ, Panicker JN, Drake M, et al. A UK consensus on the management of the bladder in multiple sclerosis. J Neurol Neurosurg Psychiatry. 2009;80:470–7.
129. McClurg D, Ashe RG, Marshall K, Lowe-Strong AS. Comparison of pelvic floor muscle training, electromyography feedback, and neuromuscular electrical stimulation for bladder dysfunction in people with multiple sclerosis. Neurourol Urodyn. 2006;25(4):337–48.
130. Alhasso AA, McKinlay J, Patrick K, Stewart L. Anticholinergic drugs versus non-drug active therapies for overactive bladder symptoms in adults. Cochrane Database Syst Rev. 2006;4:CD003193. doi: 10.1002/14651858.CD003193.pub3.
131. Mahuvrata P, Cody JD, Ellis G, Herbison GP, Hay-Smith EJC. Which anticholinergic drug for overactive bladder symptoms in adults. Cochrane Database Syst Rev. 2012;1:CD005429.
132. Fader M, Glickman S, Haggar V, Barton R, Brooks R, Malone-Lee J. Intravesical atropine compared to oral oxybutynin for neurogenic detrusor overactivity: a double-blind randomized crossover trial. J Urol. 2007;177(1):208–13.
133. Dmochowski RR, Sand PK, Zinner NR, et al. Comparative efficacy and safety of transdermal oxybutynin and oral tolterodine versus placebo in previously treated patients with urge and mixed urinary incontinence. Urology. 2003;62(2):237–42.
134. Bosma R, Wynia K, Havlikova E, de Keyser J, Middel B. Efficacy of desmopressin in patients with multiple sclerosis suffering from bladder dysfunction: a meta-analysis. Acta Neurol Scand. 2005;112(1):1–5.
135. Suchowersky O, Furtado S, Rohs G. Beneficial effect of intranasal desmopressin for nocturnal polyuria in Parkinson's disease. Mov Disord. 1995;10(3):337–40.
136. Sakakibara R, Matsuda S, Uchiyama T, Yoshiyama M, Yamanishi T, Hattori T. The effect of intranasal desmopressin on nocturnal waking in urination in multiple system atrophy patients with nocturnal polyuria. Clin Auton Res. 2003;13(2):106–8.
137. Duthie JB, Vincent M, Herbison GP, Wilson DI, Wilson D. Botulinum toxin injections for adults with overactive bladder syndrome. Cochrane Database Syst Rev. 2011;12:CD005493.
138. Khan S, Game X, Kalsi V, et al. Long term effect on quality of life of repeat detrusor injections of botulinum neurotoxin-A for detrusor overactivity in patients with multiple sclerosis. J Urol. 2011;185(4):1344–9.
139. Giannantoni A, Rossi A, Mearini E, del Zingaro M, Porena M, Berardelli A. Botulinum toxin A for overactive bladder and detrusor muscle overactivity in patients with Parkinson's disease and multiple system atrophy. J Urol. 2009;182(4):1453–7.
140. Shekelle PG, Morton SC, Clark KA, Pathak M, Vickrey BG. Systematic review of risk factors for urinary tract infections in adults with spinal cord dysfunction. J Spinal Cord Med. 1999;22(4):258–72.
141. National Collaborating Centre for Women's and Children's Health. Urinary incontinence: the management of urinary incontinence in women. London: Royal College of Obstetricians and Gynaecologists; 2006.
142. Sheriff MK, Foley S, McFarlane J, Nauth-Misir R, Craggs M, Shah PJ. Long-term suprapubic catheterisation: clinical outcome and satisfaction survey. Spinal Cord. 1998;36(3):171–6.
143. Horstink M, Tolosa E, Bonucelli U, et al. Review of the therapeutic management of Parkinson's disease. Report of a joint task force of the European Federation of Neurological Societies (EFNS) and the Movement Disorder Society- European Section (MDS-ES). Part II: late (complicated) Parkinson's disease. Eur J Neurol. 2006;13:1186–202.
144. Ahlskog JE, Muenter MD. Frequency of levodopa-related dyskinesias and motor fluctuations as estimated from the cumulative literature. Mov Disord. 2001;16(3):448–58.
145. Kumar N, Van Gerpen JA, Bower JH, Ahlskog JE. Levodopa-dyskinesia incidence by age of Parkinson's disease onset. Mov Disord. 2005;20(3):342–4.
146. Chapuis S, Ouchchane L, Metz O, Gerbaud L, Durif F. Impact of the motor complications of Parkinson's disease on the quality of life. Mov Disord. 2005;20(2):224–30.
147. Fabbrini G, Brotchie JM, Grandas F, Nomoto M, Goetz CG. Levodopa-induced dyskinesias. Mov Disord. 2007;22(10):1379–89.
148. O'Sullivan SS, Massey LA, Williams DR, et al. Clinical outcomes of progressive supranuclear palsy and multiple system atrophy. Brain. 2008;131:1362–72.

149. Crosby NJ, Deane K, Clarke CE. Amantadine for dyskinesia in Parkinson's disease. Cochrane Database Syst Rev. 2003;2:CD003467.
150. Pahwa R, Factor SA, Lyons KE, et al. Practice parameters: treatment of Parkinson's disease with motor fluctuations and dyskinesia (an evidence-based review): report of the quality standards subcommittee of the American Academy of Neurology. Neurology. 2006;66:983–95.
151. Barnes J, David AS. Visual hallucinations in Parkinson's disease: a review and phenomenological survey. J Neurol Neurosurg Psychiatry. 2001;70(6):727–33.
152. McKeith IG, Galasko D, Kosaka K, et al. Consensus guidelines for the clinical and pathological diagnosis of dementia with lewy bodies (DLB): report of the consortium on DLB international workshop. Neurology. 1996;47:1113–24.
153. McKeith IG. Dementia with lewy bodies. Br J Psychiatry. 2002;180:144–7.
154. Morgante L, Epifanio A, Spina E, et al. Quetiapine and clozapine in parkinsonian patients with dopaminergic psychosis. Clin Neuropharmacol. 2004;27(4):153–6.
155. Reading PJ, Luce AK, McKeith IG. Rivastigmine in the treatment of parkinsonian psychosis and cognitive impairment: preliminary findings from an open trial. Mov Disord. 2001; 16(6):1171–4.
156. Ezzo J, Richardson MA, Vickers A, et al. Acupuncture-point stimulation for chemotherapy-induced nausea or vomiting. Cochrane Database Syst Rev. 2006;2:CD002285.
157. Zoldan J, Friedberg G, Livneh M, Melamed E. Psychosis in advanced Parkinson's disease. Treatment with ondansetron, a 5-HT3 receptor antagonist. Neurology. 1995;45(7):1305–8.
158. Vollmer H. Comparative value of solanaceous alkaloids in the treatment of Parkinson's syndrome. Arch Neurol Psychiatry. 1942;48:72–84.
159. Barclay CL, Lang AE. Dystonia in progressive supranuclear palsy. J Neurol Neurosurg Psychiatry. 1997;62:352–6.
160. Ramasamy B, Rowe F, Freeman G, Owen M, Noonan C. Modified lundie loops improve apraxia of eyelid opening. J Neuroophthalmol. 2007;27(1):32–5.
161. Simpson DM, Blitzer A, Brashear A, et al. Assessment: botulinum neurotoxin for the treatment of movement disorders (an evidence-based review): report to the therapeutics and technology assessment subcommittee of the American Academy of Neurology. Neurology. 2008;70:1699–706.
162. Jankovic J. Pretarsal injection of botulinum toxin for blepharospasm and apraxia of eyelid opening. J Neurol Neurosurg Psychiatry. 1996;60(6):704.
163. Burn DJ, Warren NM. Towards future therapies in progressive supranuclear palsy. Mov Disord. 2005;20 Suppl 12:S92–8.
164. Swingler RJ, Compston DA. The morbidity of multiple sclerosis. Q J Med. 1992;83(300): 325–37.
165. Hickman SJ, Brierley CMH, Silver NC, et al. Infratentorial hypointense lesion volume on T1-weighted magnetic resonance imaging correlates with disability in patients with chronic cerebellar ataxia due to multiple sclerosis. J Neurol Sci. 2001;187(1–2):35–9.
166. Prosperini L, Kouleridou A, Petsas N, et al. The relationship between infratentorial lesions, balance deficit and accidental falls in multiple sclerosis. J Neurol Sci. 2011;304(1–2): 55–60.
167. Mills RJ, Yap L, Young CA. Treatment for ataxia in multiple sclerosis. Cochrane Database Syst Rev. 2007;1:CD005029.
168. Kirkwood SC, Su JL, Conneally PM, Foroud T. Progression of symptoms in the early and middle stages of Huntington's disease. Arch Neurol. 2001;58(2):273–8.
169. Andre VM, Cepeda C, Levine MS. Dopamine and glutamate in Huntington's disease: a balancing act. CNS Neurosci Ther. 2010;16(3):163–78.
170. Huntington Study Group. Tetrabenazine as antichorea therapy in Huntington's disease: a randomized control trial. Neurology. 2006;66(3):366–72.
171. Quinn N, Marsden CD. A double blind trial of sulpiride in Huntington's disease and tardive dyskinesia. J Neurol Neurosurg Psychiatry. 1984;47:844–7.
172. Mestre T, Ferreira J, Coelho MM, Rosa M, Sampalo C. Therapeutic interventions for symptomatic treatment in Huntington's disease. Cochrane Database Syst Rev. 2009;3:CD006456.

Chapter 5
Holistic Care: Psychosocial and Spiritual Aspects

Colin W. Campbell, Barbara J. Chandler, and Sue Smith

Abstract Recognizing the individual behind their disease, and "hearing their story," is the key to helping people with advanced neurological disease. Good neurological care will always require more than physical examination and inquiring about physical symptoms.

Getting to know the individual and what is important to them is essential. It also requires sensitivity and an ability to work in an equal two-way relationship. It can be a normal part of the everyday professional relationship for those in the clinical professions, but elevated professionalism with an uneven power dynamic has no part in this. Recognizing the individual's spirituality in the widest sense, and going some way to meet those needs, may be a challenge which many in the caring professions are already doing on a daily basis. A neurological illness which may affect the ability to communicate and to think rationally can easily have a deleterious effect on relationships and on sexuality. There are, however, some simple principles which can be used to help couples living with a neurological disease, particularly in the realms of sexuality.

Advanced neurological disease will impact on and often hurt those around the person with the illness, and support for partners and family should be an integral part of overall care. Expert help with financial, housing, and practical support will be required increasingly as the illness progresses. There may be many obstacles to providing care in these diseases, particularly in the more advanced phases, but there are still important and powerful ways to help these people and those who are important to them, requiring time, patience, and drawing on personal skills and attitudes.

Keywords Loss • Identity • Family • Sexuality • Spirituality

C.W. Campbell, MBChB, FRCGP, FRCP (✉)
St. Catherine's Hospice, Throxenby Lane, Scarborough YO12 5RE, UK
e-mail: colin.campbell@st-catherineshospice.org.uk

B.J. Chandler, B.Med.Sci., M.B.B.S., M.D., FRCP
Raigmore Hospital, Inverness, Scotland, UK

S. Smith, M.Sc.
Motor Neurone Disease Association, Leeds, West Yorkshire, UK

D. Oliver (ed.), *End of Life Care in Neurological Disease*,
DOI 10.1007/978-0-85729-682-5_5, © Springer-Verlag London 2013

Clinical Vignette

Cynthia J was a lady in her 60s who had MND. She had intractable problems with excess saliva, despite many attempts to resolve this. Because of embarrassing drooling in public places, she found that she could no longer meet her friends for a coffee. In effect, she no longer had a social life. This was doubly hard for her as she had been caring for a very sick husband for several years who had only recently died. She had just started to go out and meet friends again when her symptoms began. She felt that she had been cheated by her diagnosis and was struggling emotionally and socially, as was her daughter.

Reactions to Disease Progression

Introduction

The most powerful way to help someone with advanced neurological disease is to hear their concerns. Sometimes the patient's need to talk about how they are coping with their disease, and to tell their subjective version, is not always adequately heard.

"Can I ask what is the worst thing about this illness for you?" is a question which will often reveal that their greatest concern is not necessarily physical at all but rooted in the individual's psyche.

Common themes emerging from inquiries about subjective coping include:

- Not being able to do things independently
- Loss of control
- Not knowing what is going to happen
- Concern about the effect of the illness on family members

Do Psychosocial Problems Matter?

People living with progressive neurological disease may be justifiably *frightened* by many aspects of their illness. Their illness may impose numerous *threats*, including that of their ultimate survival. Many aspects of their sense of well-being may also be threatened. They may come to live too with *multiple losses*, from the ability to control their limbs, communication, continence, sexual function, and to their faculty for rational thinking.

Because the disease may progress in an apparently arbitrary and sometimes relentless fashion, they may lose their sense of *control*.

They may lose their *sense of identity*: other people may come to regard them, and treat them, differently. People may disregard who they are as individuals or who they have been prior to their illness.

This psychological maelstrom may be bubbling just behind the smiling face of the next patient, and so the approach may need to alter in order to facilitate any kind of therapeutic relationship. The stereotyped western medical model of "routine," but safe questioning, concerned only with physical functioning cannot be expected to elicit what is actually troubling the individual. The traditional obsession with eliciting neurological signs in the consulting room and on hospital scans is important. It can, however, unhelpfully promote the power of the clinician and the passiveness of the patient. Conversely, engaging in an equal two-way dialogue with the person, and sensitively inquiring what is actually of concern, may help restore a sense of control.

How Might We Respond to These Psychological Needs?

The key to establishing a therapeutic relationship with those who have progressive incurable disease is, firstly, to become acquainted with them as individuals and to "hear their agenda" [1, 2]. This is not soft, or nebulous, or just courteous. Typically, this therapeutic approach, anchored in respectful acceptance of the other, and recognizing the other's individuality, is characterized by facilitative listening.

One woman with MND described how she looked forward to meetings with members of the team caring for her and how "her spirit and well-being was greatly improved by each one" [3].

It seems that those who can engage most authentically with their patients (who in turn may be funny, or quirky, or courageous, or downright stubborn) will be in a stronger position to help that individual draw on their own strengths to deal with the challenges they face. This kind of therapeutic relationship is more about "walking alongside," listening and encouraging, facilitating and empowering. Curiously, this is the antithesis of the western medical model of the specialist doing "things" passively to the patient, even if the things are therapeutic interventions!

Clinical Vignette: A Man Who Needs to Be Heard!

James Clifford is a 54-year-old married man who was diagnosed with progressive supranuclear palsy (PSP) 2 years ago. He has had to retire from his job as sales director of a large national company. He has already sought the opinions of several different neurology specialists and has undergone repeated investigations, hoping perhaps to overturn the diagnosis. In the belief that there must be something "out there" which will help him, he is now trying a course of shark fin extract which he obtains from an unlicensed source on the Internet.

He comes to see you at your outpatient clinic, in your role as a hospital doctor. As his weary-looking wife wheels him into the room in his oversized wheelchair, he emanates aggression. He is a big man with a prominent red scratch on his face where his wife has tried to shave him. His disabling dysarthria does not disguise his message, even if it takes longer for him to express clearly what he is trying to say.

"What I need from you…what I want from you….. is a letter to say I am fit to travel. I'm going to do things my way now. I'm going to a country where at least the medics can help people like me end it all. I'll take the medicine….. and get it over with. And she agrees!"

She, Jane Clifford, the exhausted wife, is apologetic.

"He is at his wit's end, doctor, and no one seems to be listening to him."

She explains to you, later, that her life has changed out of all recognition after many good years of happy, if eventful, marriage.

You ask James, "Can I ask you, what is the worst thing about this disease for you?"

James gives you eye contact for the first time. "Not being able to do things for myself."

With no real idea what to expect, you ask him, "What would you like to see happen?"

He looks into the distance for a few seconds, then replies, "I know I can't go back to what I was… but what I want is…for people to listen to me. I want people to hear me for who I am. I am a sales director! That's who I am. Not some half-dead invalid stuck in a wheelchair. I need people to speak to me….. and not ask my wife whether 'he' wants a cup of tea!"

Issues at Diagnosis

This vignette shows various aspects of loss and change:

Loss of control: James was a powerful and successful businessman who was used to telling other people what to do. He had actually been a popular boss, and he had enjoyed a relaxed social poise in any setting, an attribute which now completely eludes him.

Loss of identity: He was used to people seeking out his opinions, and he had been unaware of how important his success had been to whom he perceived himself to be.

Fear: He is frightened of further loss of control and of his situation becoming completely intolerable to him.

Major threats: His life is going from bad to worse because of the relentless progression of his disease. This previously articulate and suave individual is struggling with dysarthria which is eroding his ability to express himself. Becoming utterly dependent on other people "doing things to him" passively, without his direction or input, is a quite unacceptable threat to him. In short, his need for control is compromised from many different threats.

Multiple losses: He has had to give up the career which was so important to the substance of whom he felt himself to be. Note that when asked what he would like to see happen, he did not allude (at this stage) to any of the problems with limb function or swallowing or intellect. His main concern was about loss of identity. He may also recognize that his relationship with his wife has altered and he is now very largely dependent on her for many of his everyday physical needs (including shaving).

Physical: ….and he has some interesting neurological signs attributable to his PSP!

Therapeutic Responses

This vignette shows various aspects of loss and change:

James' quest for assisted suicide is possibly an "insurance policy" to call a halt to his suffering at the time of his choice, if it all becomes too much to bear. In the United Kingdom, it is illegal to offer euthanasia or to help someone in any way to achieve that. This should be explained to James, with the candid recognition that you sense the desperation of his situation if things have reached that stage.

However, there are some powerful ways to start helping him. It would be useful to explore why he feels this way and allow him to express his frustrations, helplessness, and loss of control.

It may be that if James' quest for euthanasia is a vehicle for regaining control, then this is a useful *"trigger"* [4] to discuss other means of recovering control. This may be an opportunity to discuss how his illness may go on from here and to help him decide what treatment and other choices he may wish to make. He may choose to decline some of the life-prolonging treatments which may be offered to him in the future, and he will need you to guide him as to what the valid alternatives would be in those circumstances.

James may not know at this stage about the option (in the UK) of writing an advance decision to refuse treatment (ADRT) or that he could confer on his wife lasting power of attorney (LPA), giving her the power to make contemporaneous decisions about life-prolonging treatments in the future if he loses the ability to make these decisions himself.

Sharing information with the individual, in manageable portions, and when he is ready to hear them, may be an important component of returning control. Furthermore, acquiring knowledge of how his particular illness may progress in the future may be particularly important for advance care planning, especially if the illness is associated with an increasing risk of cognitive impairment.

Cognitive Change

Cognitive impairment is probably the last great taboo subject in advanced neurological disease. While it is usually acceptable to patients and families to talk about dysarthric speech, hallucinations, and even incontinence, it is often especially painful to acknowledge the presence of cognitive problems. Yet changes in the ability to think and reason normally, with the associated effects on behavior and even personality, are common in neurological diseases.

However, if cognitive impairment is present, it is important to recognize it. It can affect the person's capacity to make wise choices for themselves, making them particularly vulnerable.

Some neurological diseases particularly predispose to cognitive problems. While each disease may be associated with characteristic patterns of cognitive impairment, there is considerable scope for variation between individuals.

How Common Is Cognitive Impairment and What Form Does It Take?

Multiple Sclerosis (MS)

Overall, some degree of cognitive impairment is said to occur in up to 65 % of people with MS [5]. In one large cross-sectional study, even in patients with early disease and mild physical disability, over half had some degree of cognitive impairment on objective testing. Almost a quarter were frankly cognitively impaired.

Unfortunately too, once cognitive symptoms are established, spontaneous improvement is unusual [6]. There is an apparent association between the volume of disease on MRI scans of the nervous system and the likelihood of cognitive impairment [7].

In MS, the typical pattern of cognitive impairment is often the difficulty in learning new facts. Taking longer to process information [8] may be particularly evident in conversation and memory, and verbal fluency may be affected [8]. Formal means of assessing cognitive impairment in MS have been described [8, 9] but are not commonly used in practice.

Parkinson's Disease (PD)

There are problems with "executive" function, including planning even simple activities and following them through. Setting out the cutlery for a simple meal may assume considerable difficulties. Behavioral features with depression and apathy are also common. Hallucinations often feature prominently, although they may respond to subtle changes in medication, as dopamine-binding drugs, including levodopa, may exacerbate hallucinations [10]. Even in early PD, problems have been identified with planning and initiating activity, slowness in problem solving, and adapting to new situations [11].

Dementia in Parkinson's Disease

The incidence of dementia in PD is increased up to six times, with up to 30 % of people affected. PD-associated dementia is commoner with increasing age and with the akinetic-rigid form of the disease [10]. A key feature of PD dementia is the fact that the person has difficulty with everyday living because of cognitive deficits, independent of any other problems arising from the disease [11]. Dementia in PD is also characterized by problems with attention and memory problems. There are specific diagnostic tests to be used for PD-associated dementia [11].

Significantly, a large placebo-controlled randomized trial has shown that the dual cholinesterase inhibitor drug rivastigmine may give some improvement in mild to moderate dementia associated with Parkinson's disease [12].

Motor Neurone Disease (MND)

Historically, it was always assumed that cognitive change was very uncommon in MND. However, in one study involving 279 patients with MND, some degree of cognitive impairment (usually involving the frontal lobes) was reported in over 50 % of the patients [13]. Characteristically, problems arise with planning activities, learning new things, and using language [14]. Carers of people with MND have described self-centeredness and reduced concern for the feelings of others, while other patients were reportedly more irritable [15]. Emotional lability affects some patients, while others have blunting of emotions. Sometimes, families and even professional carers may underestimate or fail to recognize cognitive problems [16].

A small minority of people who have MND may have frontotemporal dementia prior to the onset of the physical symptoms of MND. In these cases, the dementia tends to progress particularly rapidly [17].

Progressive Supranuclear Palsy (PSP)

Cognitive changes in PSP include forgetfulness and dramatically slowed information processing speed [18]. The combination of severely slowed information processing and marked problems with executive function is characteristic of PSP and differentiates it from other dementias. Furthermore, executive dysfunction appears early in the course of the disease and is relatively severe.

How Might We Respond to Cognitive Impairment?

Recognizing the possibility of cognitive changes and eliciting this objectively is the first step. It is known too that cognitive impairment may be variable over short periods of time, sometimes even in the same day, as is commonly the case in multiple sclerosis. Such an individual may be lacking in insight, with impaired memory and verbal fluency in the morning, for instance. At some other time in the day, they may initiate topics of conversation and be alive with dry humor.

Crucially, if it is known that the particular disease puts the individual at risk of cognitive change, then discussions can be facilitated before losing mental capacity. Specifically, knowing what the person might feel about the common life-prolonging treatments may ensure that their choices are met. This may prevent professionals from subsequently "doing things to the person" passively, contrary to their actual wishes. Likewise, knowing their preferred place of care and death might enable plans to be put in place to achieve this for them.

It is important to recognize the toll which caring for a cognitively impaired patient may impose and that carers often face a distressing and isolating time. Supporting family and informal carers who may be physically and emotionally exhausted is essential – see Chap. 3. They may particularly value "time-out" away from the responsibilities of coping with the patient. Sometimes the knowledge that there will be short periods of respite care for the person with the disease may enable carers to continue in their role for longer.

Social Issues and Social Care

He received a death sentence. It felt like I had received a life sentence.

These were the words of Terri Wise, keynote speaker at the Allied Professionals Forum, International Symposium on ALS/MND, Philadelphia, December 1, 2004 [19]. Her husband was diagnosed with MND 3 days before their wedding.

Living with an advanced neurological disease affects not only the person but also their family, and the needs of everyone involved must be considered. Psychosocial care is a core component of palliative care and underpins the practice of all professionals involved. At the heart is the principle of working with the patient, family, and friends as a unit of care [19].

Psychosocial Issues

Providing palliative care support from an early stage opens access to support for the whole family and to recognition of their needs. This ensures extended family support which may continue after the death.

In many cases, the patient with neurological disease has to stop working as they enter the latter stages of their illness. Some partners too may have to stop working, at least temporarily, as the condition progresses and the person needs more care and support. For others, the partner may feel the need to continue working. In the DVD

"Live Every Day" [20] about a young man and his family living with MND, his wife Charlotte Bell says, "I have to work because we can't afford to live in this house if I don't work. We have to constantly rely on other people to do everything."

In some situations, the partner is able to take time off work and return to work following the death of their loved one. For others, depending on their employer, this may ultimately mean losing their job.

Social Care

Social care has a vital role to play in supporting people to live and die well in the place of their choosing [21].

Issues involved include:

- Accessing quality care at home
- Admission to a care facility
- Respite care
- Equipment and adaptations
- Finances and benefits

Care Services

In the UK, the benefits and health-care systems are currently undergoing significant change. Moreover, there is sometimes limited understanding of the needs of people with neurological diseases among the caring and health professionals who may be involved in providing this care. Coordination and clarity of care provision is very helpful and reduces the stresses for patients and families.

Families of people with neurological diseases have talked of their experiences of having different carers each day or night even in the last few days of life and their lack of knowledge and understanding. Exhausted family carers talked of the time taken in explaining the disease, current problems, and any equipment in use to different professional carers. Often at this time, the person with the condition is not able to speak or communicate well especially with strangers. One family member talked of it taking an hour to hand over her father's care to a different carer each evening. She was then unable to sleep as she was worried that this stranger would not understand or do things correctly and would not have sufficient knowledge.

In the UK, people who require carer support toward the end of their life are assessed by a social worker or care manager. The End of Life Care programme's "Supporting People to Live and Die Well" [21] is a framework for social care with ten objectives for providing a high-quality service at the end of life. It states clearly that health and social care requires an integrated approach in order to achieve a high quality of service. A key objective is that integrated care is centered on the person. It also recommends "an increase in the involvement of specialist palliative care social workers in working with families, commissioners, and providers of care, in order to achieve higher standards for all." Social care is a vital part of the complex network of care services needed. "Greater integration is needed across all care and support services, particularly social and health care to improve the experience of dying for the individual and those around them" [21].

> Vignette
> James was a single young man in his 40s. He was an ex-businessman who had become increasingly disabled over 2 or 3 years. He had flail arms resulting in him being able to do very little for himself. Over time, he required increasing noninvasive ventilation and ultimately invasive ventilation. His home was very unsuitable for his care needs, but initially he required only one carer. Eventually, he moved to a more suitable apartment for a disabled person. Now needing 24-hour care, he employed a team of seven personal assistants covering 24 h per day. He thoroughly enjoyed organizing this, choosing staff, and he had a very full social life. His local authority arranged a review of his social care at one point because of the great cost of his care package. He felt they would have preferred him to be admitted to a care home as this would have been easier and cheaper for them. A meeting was arranged at his home to discuss continuing health care funding. He fought his case very hard, and eventually an agreement was reached to share the cost and he maintained his personal assistants, remaining in his home until his death.

This is an excellent example of a personal budget, provided by the state, improving the quality of life of the patient and allowing him choice. In the UK, there is a move for almost everyone in need of care to have a personal budget, but careful planning and much support are needed.

Toward the end of life, as the person becomes increasingly disabled, their care and support needs will increase. This may be complicated by noninvasive ventilation, gastrostomy feeding, inability to communicate, problems with mobility, and possibly cognitive and behavioral changes. Providing care in these situations may be expensive for the family and can lead to the person being admitted into a care home, simply because it is cheaper and the care at home can no longer be afforded.

Moving into a Care Facility

Should the patient choose residential care, often because of their concern for their dependency on their family, high-quality care tends to be extremely expensive.

Much work is being done as a result of the End of Life Care Strategy [22] around workforce development and improved training for staff at all levels. This can be seen in some areas in particular where community palliative care specialist nurses are working closely with the care home sector to improve their knowledge and confidence and support them when caring for people with complex problems.

Respite Care

Access to respite care is difficult as very few hospices are able to provide this on a regular basis, and few other facilities are available. A range of imaginative high-quality respite care is needed to ensure support for everyone who needs it.

Equipment and Adaptations

A major issue regarding housing is the need for physical changes to the home. Often, people resist major adaptations, and should a Disabled Facilities Grant from the local authority be required to pay for this, it is means tested and can take many months to obtain, often arriving too late for the patient to benefit from it.

Benefits

Access to benefits in the UK is undergoing considerable change. Costs for care have increased considerably, and if the patient, and often the partner, is unable to work, this will result in a sharp drop in income at a time of greatest need. New criteria for access to benefits lean toward assuming someone can work unless proven otherwise. Affected individuals may require considerable persistence at a time when their energy is low in order to receive financial benefits. Increasingly, people have to go to a tribunal in order to receive benefits. Similarly, disability allowances are becoming more difficult to access.

Throughout the disease journey, and especially in the process of maintaining the person in the place of their choice, large numbers of different team members are needed. This may result in visits every day to the person with the neurological condition, and the family is required to retell the story and leading to confusion. The End of Life Care Strategy recommends "a key worker is appointed to avoid much duplication and confusion and achieve consistency of care for the individual" [23]. It has also been suggested that a "key-team" approach may be helpful, allowing access to team members who know of the person and family at all times and not dependent on one or two individuals [4].

Support Specifically for Families and Carers

All of the previous sections relate to both the person who is ill and their family, especially their partner, who frequently does not see him/herself as a "carer" but as a spouse, despite devoting huge amounts of time and energy to the caring role. Charlotte Bell says in the DVD [20], "we had so many plans, now it's just surviving, just getting through each day."

Evidence has shown that the use of some complex interventions such as noninvasive ventilation improves the quality of life for the patient but decreases the quality of life in almost equal measures for the carer [24]. The needs of the carer must be taken into account when introducing anything new and complex.

The End of Life Care Strategy and other related systems are in place to enable both the person nearing the end of their life and their family to get on with living too. There are numerous examples already given which show the difficulties and struggles involved, but there are also numerous examples of good practice and good support which do enable choice and dignity. Unfortunately, there is still much to do to ensure fair access to end of life and palliative care for all.

As Gallagher and Monroe state, "For most people only by being given access to palliative care are they given the opportunity to explore their feelings and understanding" [25]. They suggest "the assessment and continuing review of psychosocial concerns must recognize the particular issues faced by carers and children living with ALS. Good psychosocial care also recognizes the challenges for the professionals involved."

Opportunities are available to access support. Most of the neurological charities have local branches which serve local communities in fund raising, awareness raising, and offering social opportunities, as do the hospices and, increasingly, regional neurological alliances. There may be opportunities locally to attend "expert patient" programs. Care needs to be taken to allow their ongoing involvement toward the end of life when they may be less able to attend meetings, or yet another loss can occur. With modern social and electronic networking, this is often possible for those with the relevant computer skills and access to equipment. It can be much more difficult for those less able to use such equipment.

For carers, there may be a need for an outlet specifically aimed at them and not their partner. Some are generic local services, some run by the neurological charities, and some by hospice and palliative care services. Carers' groups are becoming more available since the advent of the National Carer Strategy [26]. There is clearly a need for more carer support throughout the disease journey and especially toward the end of the patient's life.

Children and Young People

Support for children and young people is important. Children and young people are resilient and can cope usually if they are involved, informed, and supported. Inevitably, they notice and recognize changes and these need addressing.

Vignette

One young man with MND and bulbar problems took his young daughter out to the seaside for the day. When they arrived, he took her for an ice cream and was greeted by the ice cream vendor with "you've been drinking early, haven't you?" as his voice was deteriorating. He was distraught, but the little girl was also upset and confused. She needed help to understand.

An added fear for some children (and indeed for the parents) is where a familial strain of the disease is possible, that they may also develop the disease.

Vignette

A young man recently was diagnosed with MND when his first son was just a few months old. His father and grandfather had both died from MND. His fear for his son was huge and affected the whole family, and his brother was also very fearful for himself. No one can totally allay these fears, but opportunities to share them and make plans with appropriately trained professionals can and did help this family.

Young people need to be given the information they want in appropriate age-related language and at their speed, with frequent checks about understanding. Some of the neurological charities have useful booklets and workbooks for young people which families may work through together, provided they are aware of the information and supported to do so [27]. Access to support services post bereavement for young people remains patchy across the UK. The Childhood Bereavement Network maintains a list of the services available and gives access to information to them. Access to pre-bereavement support would almost certainly be particularly helpful for those struggling with neurological conditions which will undoubtedly create changes within the home and within family relationships. Most are very locally based but Winston's Wish [28] provides some excellent written resources which may be helpful.

Recognition also needs to be given to young carers. Many young people will be helping to care for a parent or grandparent with a neurological condition who is nearing the end of their life and requiring increased support. Good palliative care assessments should ensure that these concerns will be taken into account when planning and offering support and will be able to advise and support children and young people alongside other family members.

Conclusion

Terri Wise, quoted at the beginning of this section, attempted to commit suicide when she reached the limits of her ability to cope with life. We must strive to offer quality ongoing support to everyone involved with end of life in neurological diseases.

Sexuality and Spirituality

In end of life care, the topics of sexuality and spirituality are frequently avoided because of:

- Not wanting to upset patients or relatives
- Not wanting to intrude on issues which are private and intimate
- Not wanting to cause embarrassment to self or others

The decision not to offer people an opportunity to explore these issues may deny patients and relatives a crucial aspect of holistic care. Yet the "unspoken" realms of spirituality and sexuality are both fundamental facets of human existence. Spirituality may not be recognized by the individual and may be fiercely denied when it is confused with the organized practice of religion. Sexuality is familiar to all, and yet there may be an assumption by professionals that it suddenly disappears in the face of long-term illness or disability. As one patient who had recently become a wheelchair user commented, "I have lost my femininity. There are three options in toilets when I am out: "male" (not applicable), "female" (not accessible), and "disabled." So I'm no longer feminine, I'm disabled."

Spirituality and sexuality share a common framework within holistic care, namely, the recognition of a *person*, an individual with a unique narrative [29].

Sexuality

The expression of sexuality is wide reaching. It is about self-image and self-esteem, appearance, communication, and relationships as well as sexual intimacy. It will affect the clothes we wear and the way we behave at different times and with different people. Not surprisingly, such a fundamental aspect of being human is affected by illness, but not eliminated. Within the context of end of life care, there may be a damaging and distressing assumption of, "sex will be the last thing on her mind at this stage," when intimacy within a loving relationship is just what is needed.

Sexuality and Intimate Relationships

Sexual development includes the capacity to form intimate relationships. These may be brief but for many people will be long lasting and whatever they experience in life will be in the context of this relationship. Each partner brings into a relationship:

- A set of beliefs influenced by upbringing and life experience
- Characteristic ways of behaving
- Perceptions of role
- Needs for intimacy and autonomy
- An image of self and others

Table 5.1 Some common myths associated with sexual expression [31]

Sexual activity should always lead to sexual intercourse
A man cannot be in love and fail to get an erection
Sex must be natural and spontaneous
If sex is not good, there must be something wrong with the relationship

If one partner develops an illness or disability, then the dynamics of the relationship change. For patients with neurological disease, the change may occur gradually, as with multiple sclerosis, or more rapidly in motor neurone disease, or with a frightening suddenness in acquired brain injury. Needs change with the affected partner requiring help with basic daily activities. Ideas of autonomy and the need for intimacy may change in each partner. There will be role changes within the relationship. At its most simple, who now does the shopping or manages the finances, and at a more complex interpersonal level, who initiates sexual activity? With the onset of disease or disability, the image each partner has of the other may alter. The relationship may shift from equal partners to "carer" and "cared for." Providing personal care is a parental-type role, and for the carer, expressing sexuality through physical intimacy can be difficult alongside such a role.

Common Problems, Myths, and Fears

It is only through listening to individuals that their fears and misapprehensions become apparent. A qualitative study of patients with end-stage cancer revealed that 90 % of the study participants thought sexuality should have been addressed as part of holistic care [30]. Participants felt that with the passage of time and progress of disease, emotional connection took precedence over physical expression. With regard to any form of physical expression, there were barriers within health-care settings such as shared rooms, frequent presence of staff, or size of beds. At a time of considerable loss, allowing the ongoing expression of sexuality is so important. For patients with neurological disability, whether at home or in a care setting, there are frequent intrusions: managing catheters, attending to pressure areas, help with feeding, and so on. It is so easy to forget time for intimacy and privacy with a partner. If additional care is arranged to help with some of the tasks, then that may allow time for closeness, time to be a partner rather than a carer.

There are many myths associated with sexual expression; by understanding the beliefs of individuals and couples, it may be possible to help them overcome those myths and enjoy a sexual freedom in which intimacy may be expressed whatever the limitations of illness or disability. See Table 5.1.

Approaches to Management

Acknowledging sexuality is part of holistic care, and every health and social care professional has a responsibility to recognize this area of potential stress, but not every member of the team needs to be a trained sex and relationship therapist. The *P-LI-SS-IT* model (*Permission – Limited Information – Specific Suggestions – Intensive Therapy*) may be useful as a means of enabling people to discuss sex and relationship issues [32]. It can be applied by any member of the health or social team, and it has been used as the basis of the Sex and Relationship Clinic at the Rehabilitation Centre in Newcastle and in encouraging staff to be aware of sexuality [33]. The staged approach comprises:

> *Permission* involves creating a therapeutic environment that provides "safe space" for people to raise issues that they are uncertain about. Patients may raise issues spontaneously, or an open-ended question may allow concerns to be raised. Staff are often anxious that they may be asked a question that they cannot answer, but how this is dealt with is no different for sex and relationship issues than for any other aspect of medicine. The key is to acknowledge that the patient or relative has raised an issue that is important for them and requires time to explore; and if there is no immediate answer, it can be revisited or referred to someone with more expertise. "There should be no feeling of inadequacy about not being able to give a satisfactory reply to every question asked" [34]. To ignore a question or imply that it is not relevant is unacceptable within holistic care. Seeing a couple together allows the dynamics of the relationship to be explored and may help communication. However, each partner may require an opportunity for individual discussion. Where neurological problems have affected cognition and behavior, the partner may feel they have already lost the person they knew but may not have been able to express their grief. There may be very mixed emotions in such circumstances, and only within a secure therapeutic relationship can this be discussed. Studies of couples where one has an acquired brain injury have revealed that the resultant change in behavior is potentially very damaging to intimate relationships [35]. Changes in empathy, inability to express emotion spontaneously, or lack of warmth may not be apparent to the outside world but have a profound impact on a partner [36, 37].
>
> For some people, they may not be in a relationship at this stage of their illness or they may never have had a relationship. The opportunity to reflect on experiences that were hoped for, but never happened and never will at this stage, may be very important and again require "safe space" to explore and recognize the pain of loss [34].
>
> *Limited information* is about answering questions and proactively providing information and support. Partners may be very fearful of causing pain, or of sharing emotions particularly distress, at the imminent death of their loved one. Encouraging good communication can reduce a lot of distressing anxiety. Information about managing specific symptoms to allow moments of respite and intimacy can be helpful.

Specific Suggestions

Symptom management to allow time together may involve reviewing drug schedules and fatigue management. Neuropathic pain can make areas of the body painful

Table 5.2 Spiritual and self awareness	What is important to me?
	Do I understand what is important to my patients?
	Do I respect their beliefs?
	Can I get to know this individual so I can really support them?

or uncomfortable to touch. Encouraging couples to take time to explore areas that can be stroked or massaged to give pleasure can allow an intimacy that might otherwise be missed [38]. Time together that is precious and meaningful may involve just a look, a touch, or lying down together. Partners of men with acquired brain injury coped better and experienced less stress if they had flexible coping styles [39]. If they were able to adapt and change according to need rather than trying to stick to a rigid albeit familiar pattern of life, the stress was reduced.

Intensive therapy in the form of sex and relationship therapy is rarely required, but if a couple are struggling to communicate, a brief intervention from a member of the caring team with skills either in counseling, psychology, or relationship therapy could be of great benefit. A relationship is not a static phenomenon; it changes and adapts with time, often with no need for outside help, but that help should be available if required [40].

Spirituality

End of life care rightly places great emphasis on holistic care [22]. The definition of spirit or spirituality is elusive. However, spiritual care may be easier done than described, as it is often delivered within good health care without being defined.

Spirituality is not synonymous with religion or religious practice, so although those who are part of a faith group will usually be aware of spirituality, others who are not part of a religion or faith community may be deeply spiritual. Religion is often thought to be more focused on community and practice; spirituality, separate from religious expression, is more individualist and part of an inward journey [41].

Spirituality has been defined as the essence of being, the soul, expressed through relationships to others, to the world, and within many religions, to God. However, the term spirituality may have little meaning to patients for whom concepts of spirituality may relate to narratives, relationship to self, or to nature or creativity. Indeed for health professionals, the understanding of this concept may be through daily interactions with patients and an awareness of the quest for meaning, purpose, and hope [42]. See Table 5.2.

Spirituality and Neurological Conditions

Many patients with neurological conditions have experienced multiple losses prior to the "end of life" phase of their disease. Physical disability may interfere with their ability to express their spirituality. For those belonging to a faith community, there may be difficulty in fulfilling the expected obligations of their faith. Most faiths make allowance for those who may be unable to walk unaided or unable to fulfill the demands of fasting, etc. However, despite allowances, the individual may feel great pain at no longer being able to give full expression to their faith.

For those who are not part of a faith group, there may also be losses, perhaps not being able to access a concert hall or a football ground, or simply to get out and feel the wind on their face. The problems are not only physical. Diseases such as multiple sclerosis may affect cognition and behavior and also be associated with profound fatigue. Reading which may have been a fundamental part of life may not be possible, and although talking books are good, many find they are "not the same." However, a person taking time to read to the individual may fulfill a spiritual void [43]. One patient, for whom prayer had been a central part of her life, found she no longer had the energy or attention span to pray, and potentially this could have separated her from the God of her faith and who gave meaning to her life. She started to use prayer beads, not to recite prayers but simply to hold knowing that they represented prayer and offered her a connection with what was important to her.

Spiritual Pain

Spiritual pain is often centered around loss and may be linked with psychological and physical pain but may also be quite distinct in which case analgesics and antidepressants will not help. Spiritual pain may be expressed in terms of:

- Hopelessness
- Dependency
- Altered sense of worth and isolation.

Altered cognition or communication problems may separate individuals from those around them. Recognition of distress and efforts to understand the etiology of that distress will allow help to be offered and enable the loneliness of the struggle to be alleviated. For instance, for someone with global aphasia, this may involve working to establish a means of communication, such as a blink of recognition or a meaningful squeeze of the hand. The communication may feel as if it is "one way," for example, with a patient in vegetative state. A senior nurse commented that it was impossible to nurse a patient in vegetative state without an awareness of their spirituality. This involved seeing the patient as an individual who had a history, a story to tell if they were able; this was another human being with whom to connect in that moment of caring.Not all pain can be relieved. Painful joints and dysesthesia can be relieved by medication, but the pain of loss, and unfulfilled hope, cannot simply be taken away. Providing a safe space to bear that pain and work through the issues with support as needed is one of the crucial roles of those involved in providing end of life care.

Spiritual Assessment and Provision of Spiritual Care

Within a palliative care team, hospice or hospital, there will be a chaplain or spiritual care advisor who can provide both support for the staff and for patients and relatives.

The chaplain should not be seen as the sole provider of spiritual care but as a skilled resource within the multidisciplinary team. However, many neurological patients may not have contact with a palliative care team and recognition of spiritual need, and delivery of care may lie with the health and social care team. Those patients who belong to a faith community will have access to their own faith leaders who may well offer guidance to staff in relation to patterns of spiritual expression. But if none of that is applicable, we must simply give the care that underpins our work in the "caring professions." Simply offering a greeting as one human being to another, rather than as a "professional," greeting a "patient," or a "carer" greeting the "cared for," is a step along the way. Offering a greeting whether or not it can be reciprocated physically or verbally establishes a relationship, which is the foundation of spiritual care. There are assessment tools, but a more intuitive approach using the interpersonal skills that are part of effective health care may be more discerning and more empathetic which allows the assessment process to be in itself therapeutic [44].

Spiritual Care at the End of Life

At the end of life, there are tasks that people may want to complete such as healing broken relationships, saying goodbye to those they love, letting go of future plans, and putting things in order. There may be anger that needs expressing, regrets to be shared, and fears to be acknowledged, but this assumes cognition and communication which may not be open to our neurological patients. As health and social care professionals, we form one-to-one relationships with our patients and offer an unconditional positive regard [45]. This is the bedrock of spiritual care. Professionals will find it easier to give spiritual care if they have an awareness of their own spirituality, that which gives meaning within their lives and also their own prejudices and beliefs. There is no place for proselytizing. A patient may be able to give their own narrative, but if not it is important to find out as much as possible:

- Did the individual belong to a faith community?
- What made them smile?
- What was central in their life?
- What did they do in times of celebration or sorrow?
- What had life been like?
- What losses, sadness, and joy had filled their life?

From the "patient" emerges a person with whom to connect and spiritual care begins.

Conclusion

The holistic care of the person with a neurological disease and their family will encompass a broad assessment of psychological, social, and spiritual aspects. Their own particular concerns must be heard as they are seen as individuals in their own right. In this way, they can be helped to maintain their quality of life and their relationships together.

References

1. Kritjanson LJ, Toye C, Dawson S. New dimensions in palliative care: a palliative approach to neurodegenerative diseases and final illness in older people. Med J Aust. 2003;179:S41–3.
2. Anderson PM, Borasio GD, Dengler R, et al. EFNS task force on management of amyotrophic lateral sclerosis: guidelines for diagnosing and clinical care of patients and relatives. Eur J Neurol. 2005;12:921–8.
3. Sackett B, Sakel M. A patient's journey. Motor neurone disease. BMJ. 2011;342:1025–7.
4. National End of Life Care Programme. End of life care in long term neurological conditions – a framework for implementation. 2010. http://www.endoflifecareforadults.nhs.uk/assets/downloads/neurology_report___final___20101108_1.pdf. Accessed 17.4.12.
5. Amato MP, Zipoli V, Portaccio E. Multiple sclerosis-related cognitive changes: a review of cross-sectional and longitudinal studies. J Neurol Sci. 2006;245:41–6.
6. Kujala P, Portin R, Ruutiainen J. The progress of cognitive decline in multiple sclerosis. A controlled 3-year follow-up. Brain. 1997;120:289–97.
7. Patti F, Amato MP, Trojano M, et al. Cognitive impairment and its relationship with disease measures in mildly disabled patients with relapsing-remitting multiple sclerosis: baseline results from the Cognitive Impairment in Multiple Sclerosis (COGIMUS) study. Mult Scler. 2009;15:779–88.
8. Rao SM, Leo GJ, Bernardin L, Unverzagt F. Cognitive dysfunction in multiple sclerosis. I. Frequency, patterns and prediction. Neurology. 1991;41:685–91.
9. Amato MP, Ponziani G, Siracusa G, Sorbi S. Cognitive dysfunction in early-onset multiple sclerosis: a reappraisal after 10 years. Arch Neurol. 2001;58:1602–6.
10. Emre M, Aarsland D, Brown R, et al. Clinical diagnostic criteria for dementia associated with Parkinson's disease. Mov Disord. 2007;22:1689–707.
11. Dubois B, Burn D, Goetz C, et al. Diagnostic procedures for Parkinson's disease dementia: recommendations from the movement disorder society task force. Mov Disord. 2007;22:2314–24.
12. Emre M, Aarsland D, Albanese A, et al. Rivastigmine for dementia associated with Parkinson's disease. N Engl J Med. 2004;351:2509–18.
13. Ringholz GM, Appel SH, Bradshaw M, et al. Prevalence and patterns of cognitive impairment in sporadic ALS. Neurology. 2005;65:586–90.
14. Lomen-Hoerth C, Murphy J. The neuropsychology of amyotrophic lateral sclerosis. In: Brown RH, Swash M, Pasinelli P, editors. Amyotrophic lateral sclerosis. 2nd ed. Abingdon: Informa UK; 2006.
15. Gibbons ZC, Richardson A, Neary D, et al. Behaviour in amyotrophic lateral sclerosis. Amyotroph Lateral Scler. 2008;9:67–74.
16. Lomen-Hoerth C. Characterisation of amyotrophic lateral sclerosis and fronto- temporal dementia. Dement Geriatr Cogn Disord. 2004;17:337–41.
17. Lillo P, Hodges JR. Frontotemporal dementia and motor neurone disease: overlapping clinic-pathological disorders. J Clin Neurosci. 2009;16(9):1131–5.
18. Litvan I. Cognitive disturbances in progressive supranuclear palsy. J Neural Transm. 1994;42:69–78.
19. All Party Parliamentary Group on Motor Neurone Disease. Inquiry into access to specialist palliative care for people with motor neurone disease. 2011.
20. Live Every Day [DVD] Northampton. MND Association. 2006. http://mndassociation.org/publicationslist. Accessed 15 Aug 2011.

21. National End of Life Care Programme. Supporting people to live and die well: a framework for social care at the end of life. 2010.
22. Department of Health. NHS End of Life Care Strategy. London: Department of Health; 2008.
23. Royal College of Nursing. Route to success: the key contribution of nursing to end of life. 2011.
24. Mustafa N, Walsh E, Bryant V. The effect of non invasive ventilation on ALS patients and their caregivers. Neurology. 2006;66:1211–7.
25. Gallagher D, Monroe B. Psychosocial care in palliative care. In: Oliver D, Borasio GD, Walsh D, editors. Amyotrophic lateral sclerosis. Oxford: Oxford University Press; 2006.
26. Department of Health. Carers at the heart of the twenty first century; families and communities, a caring system on your side, a life of your own. London: Department of Health; 2008.
27. When someone close has MND – a workbook for children aged four to ten. Northampton: MND Association; 2009.
28. Stokes JA. Then, now and always. Cheltenham: Winston's Wish; 2004.
29. Jaramillo DM. Julie's bath. Nursing. 2004;34:61.
30. Lemieux L. Sexuality in palliative care: patient perspectives. Palliat Med. 2004;18:630–7.
31. Spence S. Psychosexual therapy: a cognitive behavioural approach. London: Chapman & Hall; 1991. p. 43.
32. Annon JS. The behavioural treatment of sexual problems: brief therapy. New York: Harper & Row; 1976.
33. Chandler BJ. Sex and relationships in neurological disability. In: RJ G, editor. Handbook of neurological rehabilitation. Hove: Psychology Press; 2003. p. 307–8.
34. Wells P. No sex please, I'm dying. A common myth explored. Eur J Polit Res. 2002;9(3): 119–22.
35. Lezac M. Living with the characterologically altered brain injured patient. J Clin Psychiatry. 1978;39:592–9.
36. Wood RL, Liossi C, Wood L. The impact of head injury neurobehavioural sequelae on personal relationships: preliminary findings. Brain Inj. 2005;19:845–51.
37. Wood R, Williams C. Inability to empathize following traumatic brain injury. J Int Neuropsychol Soc. 2008;14:289–96.
38. Ward-Abel N. Sexuality and MS: a guide for women. Hertfordshire: MS Trust; 2007.
39. Ponsford J, et al. Long term adjustment of families following TBI where comprehensive rehabilitation has been provided. Brain Inj. 2003;17:453–68.
40. Cort E. Couples in palliative care. Sex Relation Ther. 2004;19:337–54.
41. Collicutt J. Psychology, religion and spirituality. Psychologist. 2011;24(4):250–1.
42. Edwards A. The understanding of spirituality and the potential role of spiritual care in end of life and palliative care: a meta-study of qualitative research. Palliat Med. 2010;24(8):753–70.
43. Paul C. The relentless therapeutic imperative. BMJ. 2004;329:1457–9.
44. Watson MS, et al. Chapter 9: Spiritual care. In: Oxford handbook of palliative care. Oxford: Oxford University Press; 2009. p. 750–751.
45. Mearns D, Thorne B. Person centred counselling in action. London: Sage; 1999.

Chapter 6
Multidisciplinary Care

David Oliver and Sally Watson

Abstract The multidisciplinary approach to care is essential in the care of a person with a progressive neurological disease. This needs to be carefully coordinated to ensure that the various members of the team provide their own expertise and knowledge in collaboration with other team members so that the quality of life of patient and family can be maintained as effectively as possible.

For a person with a neurological disease, there may be several different teams involved, and there is an even greater need to ensure that there is close collaboration and the goals of care are shared and appropriate. The care may also engender stresses and conflicts between teams and team members, and these issues need to be recognized and addressed if the care provided is to be effective. Stresses may also be seen from the issues raised in the person's care, and all team members should be aware of the need to address these issues.

Keywords Team working • Effectiveness • Communication • Collaboration

D. Oliver, B.Sc., FRCP, FRCGP (✉)
Consultant in Palliative Medicine and Honorary Reader,
Wisdom Hospice, High Bank, Rochester, Kent ME1 2NU, UK

Centre for Professional Practice, University of Kent,
Chatham, UK
e-mail: drdjoliver@googlemail.com

S. Watson, M.A., Ph.D.
Director of Executive Education,
Lancaster University Management School,
Lancaster, Lancashire, UK
e-mail: sally.watson@lancaster.ac.uk

D. Oliver (ed.), *End of Life Care in Neurological Disease*,
DOI 10.1007/978-0-85729-682-5_6, © Springer-Verlag London 2013

Case Vignette

John was a 65-year-old man with motor neuron disease. He was married with two daughters who lived nearby with their families. He was diagnosed with motor neuron disease when he started to have problems walking and developed slurred speech. He had been attending a neurology department for 6 months before the diagnosis was finally made and had been supported by the consultant neurologist and the specialist MND nurse. At home, he was seen by his general practitioner and the community nurse, and he was referred to the local hospice team for support. He was visited by the community team and saw the consultant in palliative medicine and the clinical nurse specialist, physiotherapist, occupational therapist, and speech and language therapist visited from the rehabilitation team, and it was suggested that he saw the consultant in rehabilitation medicine.

His family was overwhelmed by the visits and all the professionals involved and became angry and did not respond to telephone messages. The hospice team agreed to coordinate the professional input, and the various teams met away from John's house and agreed that the hospice community team and GP would provide ongoing support and call on the other teams for specific help. John and his family agreed to this, and he was supported at home, with the appropriate help and equipment until his death 12 months later.

The care of a person, with a progressive neurological disease, is often complex and involves many different professionals from both health and social care. A team approach is essential, so that there is a coordinated approach and the professionals work together for the benefit of the patient and family. In the UK, the involvement of a multidisciplinary team has been emphasized in the National Service Framework for Long Term Conditions [1] – which suggests a "holistic, integrated interdisciplinary team approach to care" and the NICE Guidance on supportive and palliative care which states that the evidence "strongly supports specialist palliative care team working" [2]. In the long-term care of a patient with a neurological disease, there may be an increased complexity as several different teams may be involved, including specific services such as neurology and rehabilitation and more generalist services such as palliative care and primary care. This chapter aims to consider the evidence and research on team working and relate this to the approach to the care of patients and families.

Within many services, there appears to be little understanding and a lack of clarity of the roles and complexity of a multidisciplinary team approach. Conceptual models do suggest that a team may be seen merely as a group of people – a group being defined merely by the "presence of a social structure" of status and relationships [3]. Groups may have a collective identity, communication within the group, shared aims and objectives, a developing structure, and rules and norms which may or may not be adhered to [3]. This may give the impression of a team working together, whereas the reality may be merely a group of individuals interacting as they see fit and when they wish to.

However, over the past few years, there has been an emphasis on the development of multidisciplinary teams which can be defined as "a small number of people with complementary skills who are committed to a common purpose, performance goals, and approach for which they hold themselves mutually accountable" [4]. A common purpose and approach is especially important in multidisciplinary teams involved in the care of people over a longer period of time. There are various models of multidisciplinary teams, including:

- Multidisciplinary – each team member contributes their expertise independent of the others and all team members have their own clearly defined place. Information is provided from all team members but the final decision making leading to the treatment decision may be taken by only one member [5]. For instance, in mental health services, there may be several workers from different disciplines, who meet the patient independently, meet together to discuss issues, but the final decision may remain with the psychiatrist.
- Interdisciplinary – when a common decision making process is taken. It has been defined as "an identified collective in which members share common goals and work interdependently in planning, problem solving, decision making, and implementing and evaluating team-related tasks" [6]. For instance, in an operating theater, all the people involved in the care of the patient are dependent on each other and react together to cope with any crises that may develop.

However, teams may in fact be changing all the time – responding to the particular needs of the person and to the changes within the general population, the expectations of the public and national and local reorganizations. As the patient's needs may vary over time, the professionals involved in their care may change. This may be within the team which is most involved in the care, but may require the coordination with other teams. Thus there is a need for flexibility in who is involved but with a clarity of which professionals are or are not involved and taking responsibility for the overall care. The need for an improved multidisciplinary approach was emphasized during the care of someone with Parkinson's disease in the report of the Parkinson's Disease Society. The report suggested that "the care of people with PD is best undertaken in a multidisciplinary way throughout each stage of the disease" to reduce the problems that are encountered if there are many different professionals involved, giving potentially conflicting advice [7].

One of the potential issues facing a team is the confusion as to how the team is working and a lack of understanding of the roles within the team of the various team members. This again leads to confusion and less than optimum care for the patient and family. Criteria have been suggested which indicate that a high-performance team is working well:

- An accurate assessment in a timely manner
- Effective and integrated care
- Allow a combined approach which may achieve more than the sum of the individuals working on their own
- The interaction and the combination of skills the individuals may develop allows an approach that the individuals will not have by themselves
- Effective communication within the team, with other professionals, and with the patient and family
- Encourage audit of the team's activities and outcomes [5]

The effective team can be seen to have clarity in how they work – in the knowledge they have of the patients and each other and how they work in a collaborative way.

Team Knowledge

As the situation of the patient and family, within the wider health and social economy, is changing and the involvement of teams and their members changes continually, a continuity of knowledge of the issues and the patient is essential. The people involved within a team will have varying knowledge of the situation – the issues affecting the patient, their wishes, the roles and influences of others in this situation, including the family, and the feelings engendered by these issues. This knowledge needs to be shared within the team but this may not always be as straightforward as the team thinks as there are differing aspects of knowledge:

- The individual knowledge possessed by each team member separately – i.e., the knowledge each team member has
- The knowledge pool – the total pool of knowledge possessed by the team collectively, accounting for overlap – see Fig. 6.1
- The knowledge configuration – the varying proportions of the knowledge pool shared in common, i.e., understanding what is common knowledge and what is unique to particular team members
- Knowledge acquisition – every team member will gain knowledge at a different rate to others and this may affect the team's learning
- Knowledge emergence within the team – how the knowledge pool and configuration changes over time
- Knowledge emergence between teams – there will be differences in rates of knowledge variability, pool, and configuration across the different teams involved [8].

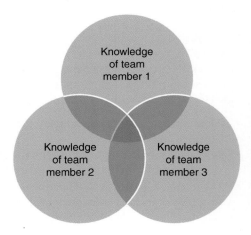

Fig. 6.1 Knowledge configuration

Often teams do not realize that their own team members have varying knowledge and awareness of the issues facing the patient, and it is assumed that "everyone knows" of changes and challenges. This is an even greater issue when different teams are involved – with very different roles and involvement – and the care provided may be confusing to all concerned. Although everyone may be aiming to improve the quality of life and care for the patient and family, this may not be achieved and they are left with mixed messages and confusion.

Team Effectiveness

In considering the most appropriate model for a multidisciplinary team caring for neurological patients, the model of team effectiveness suggested by Beckhard may be useful. He suggests that for a team to be effective, it must do more than merely share information [9]. He suggested that there were several dimensions affecting the behavior and purposes of a team, as shown in Fig. 6.2.

All these dimensions need to be considered together. Often one area is looked at, such as looking at the processes within the team, rather than ensuring that all team members are aware why that particular process or procedure is important as it leads to the ultimate goal. If the team can discuss and agree on the goal, they can then look at the processes that lead to this.

Other team approaches also stress the need for communication and clarity in purpose. Carroll et al. suggest the need to develop "collaboration competence" [10]. They suggest four realms of collaborative skills that need to be developed:

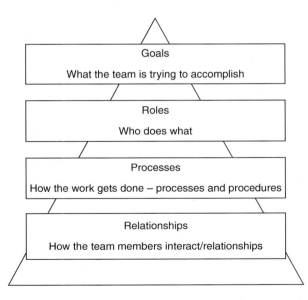

Fig. 6.2 Team effectiveness

- Planning

    This involves the development of an understanding of the goals (both explicit and implicit), the resources, and the people to enable the team to find the most appropriate and successful strategies and actions. The team should work together in an equitable way, and decisions and planning are made jointly, with no one person controlling these decisions. In this way, a shared understanding, with clarity of who will be involved, who is responsible for certain actions and the logistical aspects of the development of the plan are clear.

- Communication

    All team members participate equally, contribute ideas, and listen and understand ideas from each other and come to a shared understanding.

- Critical evaluation

    All points of view and ideas are considered in a critical and constructive way so that the final agreement is for the best ideas and actions.

- Productivity

    Careful monitoring of the plans and developments, together with adjusting to meet the changing environment and ensuring good communication and critical evaluation, aids the team to work more effectively and efficiently.

    These theoretical approaches may allow teams to look at their functioning and see ways of developing the team approach and thus maximizing the work undertaken. There will be the need for continual reassessment and change, particularly in times of national and local change, reorganization, and uncertainty. There is also the need to ensure that there is greater appreciation of the various roles and pressures within the team.

Team Appreciation of Members

Although each member has their own distinct and necessary role, it is important that they see themselves as one "instrument" within the interdisciplinary "orchestra" [5]. This includes having the confidence and skills to help in the team assessment and also to have appreciation and understanding of the roles and expertise of other team members. There needs to be a shared knowledge and understanding of roles to communicate efficiently and effectively.

The attitudes of team members – to each other and the team itself – must be considered, and the interpretation of team working is just as important as other organizational and team dynamic aspects in ensuring the team works effectively [11]. Different attitudes to teamwork have been suggested:

- A directive philosophy – based on a hierarchy where one person takes the lead on the basis of status and power.
- Integrative philosophy – all members are seen as equal and team players, and discussions within the team are seen as vital.
- Elective philosophy – team roles are seen as clear and distinct, and team members operate autonomously and only relate to each other when they feel this is necessary [11].

Within multidisciplinary teams caring for neurological patients, there may be differing views as to the team philosophy. For instance, there may be a medical member, such as the consultant, who assumes the lead whereas other team members would aim to work in a more integrated way. If these differing views of the philosophy of the team are not recognized, there can be profound conflicts, and there is need for clarity of tasks and roles within the team, together with a clear philosophy of the team dynamics.

Team Member Roles

The role within a team encompasses both the expectations of the team member and what is also expected from others in the team. There may be ambiguity within the team, and often there is overlap, which needs to be negotiated [5]. Team members may be able to develop their own skills, while acknowledging the limits of their ability, so that they can pass onto other team members, who may have more experience or particular skills that can be of help [12]. Team members may offer general support with mutual accountability so that the care provided can be clear and continuous [12].

Roles may be:

- Professional – related to professional identity but with clarity of overlap and mutual involvement
- Personal – related to the member as a person
- Formal – clearly defined role within the team, such as leader
- Informal – reflecting their particular role within the team, such as "clown" or "peacemaker"

These roles may overlap and change from day to day and from patient to patient. Team members may move in and out of differing roles, according to the situation or to the dynamics within the team. Moreover, a member may choose the role or have this allocated to them, leading to conflict with other team members or feelings of regret, frustration, or anger. If a team is to work effectively, there is a need for these roles to be clear and all team members to be aware of their own role, in association with the other team members. The team leader will enable these discussions and ensure that there is clarity and flexibility in how team members take on differing roles, in response to the patient and family and changing circumstances for the team.

Leadership

Within any team, there is the need for clear leadership to enable the team to function effectively. The leader should be defined and should guide the team by

- Keeping purpose, goals, and approach relevant and meaningful
- Building commitment and confidence of the team and its members
- Strengthening the skills of members
- Working to minimize external obstacles and managing relationships externally
- Creating opportunities for all team members to work effectively
- Ensuring that there is team cohesion and understanding to allow effectiveness
- Coping with conflicts within the team – particularly in relation to changing roles of team members

There are different theories regarding leadership:

- Strategic – developing a clear strategy and facilitating team members to work for a specific outcome
- Transformational – encouraging members to identify with the task and goals, with the formation of a shared vision
- Functional – clearly aiming to get things done and looking at the team to develop plans and negotiate activities
- Shared leadership – all team members engage as the leader with a shared understanding and consensus of the team members' expertise. There is also the need for trust of a team member who takes on the leadership role for a particular task.

Teams involved in the care of people with neurological disease may have a clearly defined leader, but the leadership role is often not clearly understood. It is important to define the way the team is to work and to be led.

However, with this patient group, it may need to be clear for someone to have overall responsibility for decision making and that the team is "not a democracy" [13]. This particularly applies when decisions may be made for a patient who has lost capacity to make the decision themselves. The UK Mental Capacity Act places the final decision in the patients' "best interests" onto the medical clinician who has overall responsibility for that patient's care – usually the general practitioner or the consultant [14]. The decision maker should take into consideration the views of the patient – if they can express them or have provided details of their wishes in an advance decision or statement – the close family, and the other members of the team involved. All team members should be involved in contributing to the decisions – defining the issues, identifying solutions, prioritizing, choosing alternatives, agreeing a time frame, and closely involving patient and family in the decision making process. Although the aim is to be "patient centered" and to allow patient choice in certain circumstances, a "best interests" decision may be necessary, and the physician will be responsible for this. This may be particularly challenging to the team as this final decision will need to be taken by the physician, with the involvement, but not necessarily the complete agreement of the rest of the team and the team. However, the final decision is theirs, and they take responsibility for this. Clear decision making and clear leadership will enable full discussion within the team, and clear communication is essential amongst all the team.

Communication

For a team to be effective, there needs to be good communication among all the team members and with the other people involved – within the family and other professional teams. This ensures that there is clarity of the aims and plan of care and all are involved in decision making. Communication is enhanced by regular, structured meetings, to allow discussion, assessment, and evaluation of patient care together with close working relationships and common records [5]. The development of a common aim and the need to evaluate the quality of care, rather than just the numbers of patients seen, will enhance team development and performance [13].

If communication is not good, then different professionals may give potentially conflicting advice to the patient and family. Patients and carers may also feel that they are asked for the same information on many occasions, if communication within the team is inadequate and team members do not use or trust information gained by others within the team. Although time-consuming, communication with all involved is helpful and reduces confusion and increases effective care.

Coordination of Care

For the patient and family, coordination of care is paramount – they do not want to repeat the same story to all professionals that they meet, and there can be confusion if they receive conflicting advice from different professionals. Moreover, many professionals may come into a person's house – general practitioner, community nurses, physiotherapist, speech and language therapist, neurology specialist nurses, specialist palliative care team members, care assistants, and social worker to say nothing of family and friends – and this can be very difficult for the patient and family as they may feel that they are losing control of the situation and find it hard to maintain their own dignity and privacy.

The concept of a "key worker" has been suggested as a way of overcoming some of these issues. This key worker would be the professional who would help to coordinate the involvement of other team members, and other professionals who may become involved in care, and would be the first contact point for the patient and family. There may be anxiety and confusion over which professional to contact if there is a problem, particularly in an emergency situation, and this can lead to unnecessary hospital admission as in the last result an ambulance is called. The key worker concept would seem to be an answer to the issue, but if this is just one individual, there can be an even greater risk of confusion and anxiety – as they will not necessarily be available 24 hours a day, 7 days a week, and throughout the year – as they will be off duty, annual leave, and sickness. It may be easier for the patient and family if there is a single point of contact, with a larger team with knowledge about the issues for the patient and a willingness to help and advise.

This concept of a "key team" was emphasized by a working party in the UK, exploring the interfaces between neurology, rehabilitation, and palliative care. They suggested that

"Neurology, rehabilitation and palliative care services should develop closely co-ordinated working links to support people with long-term neurological conditions from diagnosis to death, including:

- A proper flow of communication and information for patients and their families
- A designated point of contact for each stage in the pathway
- A needs assessment identifying the patient's individual problems" [15].

Services need to be tailored to suit individual needs and professionals need to be sensitive to those aspects of life that remain important and central to the individual and their family. The difficulties of multiprofessional involvement can be surmounted by good communication and a clear point of contact for the individual and their family. This may need to be with a specific team – so that contact is not dependent on a specific team member – and advice and support is always available. This will help to ensure that there is always the opportunity for support at all times.

Multiple Teams/Multiple Problems

The number of professionals involved with one individual and their family will vary at different points on the patient journey and may be greatest for patients with advanced disease, when the individual may have the least energy for coordinating their care. Families may also be experiencing the exhaustion and stress of their caring role, and the added burden of trying to coordinate professional contacts can be overwhelming. Decisions that will affect the end of life care of the individual may be discussed at this time, and it essential that there is an established, reliable means of communication between professionals, coordinating their involvement and communication with the individual patient and all those involved in the care of that patient and their family.

Throughout the patient journey, there may be different teams collaborating in the care:

- At the time of diagnosis, the GP and neurologist.
- As the disease progresses, specialist neurological nurses and other professionals to assess specific needs – physiotherapist, occupational therapist.
- With increasing difficulties new teams – a person with MND may meet a respiratory team for assessment of respiratory function and consideration of respiratory support or a gastroenterology team for assessment and consideration for gastrostomy placement and feeding.

- As the disease advances, there may be palliative care/hospice teams involved, together with increasing community support, including community nursing and care support.
- At the end of life, specialist palliative care teams, including new team members.

This varying team interaction and collaboration can cause even greater confusion to patients and families and also to all the professionals involved. The professional needs to be aware of the complexity of the situation and aim to reduce the numbers of people contacting the patient and family and to coordinate the care, if possible through the key team.

There may also be issues of differences in the goals, roles, processes, and relationships within the different teams. There may be shared goals in the overall care of the patient and family, but these may not always be clear to all teams and their members. Moreover, there will be overlap and interaction between teams and the team members which may lead to confusion to the patient, conflict, and poor outcomes. This complexity is represented in Fig. 6.3.

The complexity of all the relationships is clear in Fig. 6.3, and the need for close collaboration can be clearly seen. Moreover, the need for discussion and clarification

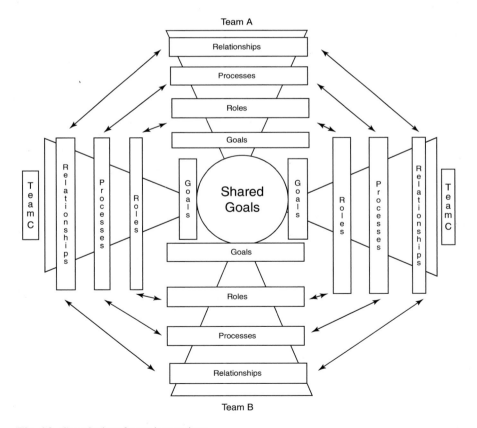

Fig. 6.3 Complexity of team interactions

of role and processes and development of relationships can be seen if common goals are to be developed and then acted upon. Although each team may have its own goals, it is important for a coordinated team approach to develop common goals, with the involvement of all the teams with the patient and family. This may be difficult, particularly if there are conflicts between the goals of the various teams, and careful discussion and planning may be necessary.

In health and social care, it is not always clear that these discussions and awareness of the needs to look at all aspects of care do occur. There is the risk of increasing complexity of the systems with the changes in the NHS in the UK as there may be increasing local development and involvement of charities and independent services, including for profit companies. It is becoming increasingly important to develop clear pathways of care with clear goals. However, this will need to be supported by close collaboration and discussion between the various teams involved so that all areas are considered – relationships, processes, roles, and goals – if patient care is to be provided in an efficient and appropriate way for the benefit of patients and their families.

Communication Between Multiple Teams

Communication is essential so that all involved are aware of changes and plans. Meetings may be helpful, and documentation, which can remain with the patient and be added to by any professional seeing the patient, should be used to record activities, actions, and plans. The factors to be considered include:

- What information do my colleagues need – and what would I appreciate receiving myself?
- What is the management plan?
- Is everyone clear as to their responsibilities?
- How do we continue the communication? [16]

Commitment to communicate and ease these issues is essential from all involved, for if the professionals are unclear, the patient and family are at risk of increasing confusion and anxiety. All teams need to respect other teams and their members, and if there appear to be conflicts, these should be raised with the professionals involved, and certainly not in front of the patient and family, who need to be reassured that there is a team approach and that they can have confidence in the coordinated care [16].

This key team approach can be very helpful as the patient and family know who they may contact if they have concerns, and that when the contact is made, they will be known and their concerns listened to and understood so that the appropriate action can take place. Moreover, the various teams and professionals are also aware of the contact point so that they are able to obtain information and respond appropriately. This coordinated approach should continue at all times, and increasingly, there are locality-based registers of people with long-term neurological conditions, or at the end of life, so that all professionals can obtain basic information on the person's care and preferences and the teams involved.

Team Conflict

There may be areas of conflict develop when goals are considered. In these changing times, there are increasing challenges to teams both in health and social care. There is a tendency for organizations – nationally and locally – to develop standards as goals and different team members may see these in different ways. Although outcome measures are seen as important, they are often measurements of process – such as the number of visits or contacts with patients – that do not reflect the complexity of working with people with progressive disease. Careful consideration and clarification of the goals may allow the processes and measurement of the process/pathway to be clearer and feel more appropriate for the professionals involved. However, on occasions, teams may be faced with complex processes and procedures that seem to conflict with their professional aims of working with patients and families to improve quality of life and meet their particular needs. This conflict cannot be overcome easily, especially if this is firmly a national directive, but the team can at least ensure that they are all aware of the issues and come to an agreement of the best way of coping with these conflicts.

There are many areas in team working that may lead to conflict – within the team, with patients and families, or with other professional teams:

- Ambiguous boundaries
- Interdisciplinary rivalry
- Communication barriers
- Leadership not meeting the team needs
- Decision making excluding some team members
- Different expectations goals between members
- Previous conflicts leading to displaced hostility
- Different personality styles
- Continuing change threatening roles of team members or team itself
- Scarcity of resources [12]

A well-functioning team, with good leadership, may be able to preempt these issues and ensure that any conflicts are identified and addressed quickly, before long-term damage occurs. All team members are responsible for ensuring that conflict and stresses are identified, and time is needed within the team for consideration of these issues.

The consideration of conflicts and team development should also be part of all team meetings, allowing reflection on work-related issues and the dynamics within the team [12]. This will enable a degree of safety and trust within the team to allow honest and constructive discussion, leading to a resolution of the issues raised [12]. On occasions, with complex issues, there may be the need for external facilitation. Clinical supervision

– "a formal process of professional support and learning which enables individual practitioners to develop knowledge and competence, assume responsibility for their own practice and enhance consumer protection and safety of care in complex clinical situations" [17] – has been recognized as a tool to support teams preventing and resolving team conflicts. Clear and supportive supervision can help in building the team itself and facilitate development of not only each team member but the team itself.

Team building can be ongoing in everyday practice [18]. It has been suggested that there is a positive attitude to resolving issues as and when they arise and to develop an approach which encourages difficulties and potential conflicts to be raised and considered:

- Agreeing general rules of behavior between team members, especially when there are differences in power and status
- Agreeing when and how difficult issues should be resolved
- Identifying and trying to resolve uncertainties and barriers to communication or work flow
- Giving priority to sorting out issues, particularly when team members have to deal with each other frequently or where there is a history of conflict and difficult relationships [18]

Frequent review of the care provided is also important to look at and evaluate the team's activities – this may be with regular case discussion, after-event reviews following a significant event or error, or review of times when communication or decision making has been particularly difficult [18]. This allows regular assessment of team functioning and the opportunity for improvement and minimizing conflict. This same review is also essential for the collaboration and interaction between teams.

Team Stress and Pressures

All teams face problems and have to cope with difficult interactions and stresses. These may include:

- Conflicts between team members
- Conflicts between the multiple teams that may be involved in the person's care
- Relationship issues between team members

    Specifically related to team working
    Related to the team members themselves

        Specific issues for their own role
        Home and health issues that may be affecting their capacity to work effectively

- The intense emotions that may arise in caring for people with increasing disability and facing deterioration and death.

Team Resilience

Teams need to develop resilience, which may be defined as "unpredicted and markedly successful adaptations to negative life events, trauma, stress, and other forms of risk" [19]. Resilience assumes that there will be stresses and adversity – and things will not always go well [18]. It has been suggested that consideration of the theories of resilience would be helpful in considering the developing relationships within teams – as team members will be affected by their past experiences of close relationships when they work closely together, particularly with complex and stressful client groups [18].

Team Identity

Teams face many issues regarding identity which can lead to stress within the team – which may conflict or challenge the person's own concept of their own identity. This may include, but is not limited to, gender, faith, and nationality but will also include issues regarding:

- Professional identity
- Personal loyalty to other team members
- Personal, family , community roles, and commitments
- Work group identity with differing views within the team [18]

Teams need to consider these issues and ensure that there are clear ways of resolving conflict early so that ongoing resentment and conflict do not develop.

Team Challenges

Teams will also face adversities – situations that may be difficult to adapt to, as individuals, teams, or organizations:

- Individual team members

  Their own psychological makeup and the way they react as an individual
  Their own home circumstances and the stresses they may face within their own relationships or families

- Teams themselves

  Structures and policies that may cause conflict with team members' own standards and ethical stance, such as altering care pathways under the influence of commissioning services

- Organizations or society

  Funding or changes within the wider organization, such as reorganization affecting future plans and developments
  Policy makers within the wider society – both political structures or changes in health and social care – may lead to increased stress. Wider society norms may change and affect the team function, such as legal changes affecting care, for instance, changes in immigration rules or the legislation of assisted suicide in a country.

- Patients

  Patients will be facing their own stresses, which may be related to their condition and deteriorating condition, or be separate from these – such as bereavement, marital distress, divorce, housing, or financial changes.

As well as considering these stressors, it is important to consider the way in which team members react to them. One individual may be affected first, and the adversity flows through the team, creating different emotional reactions which may reduce or heighten both the flow and the adversity. There need to be clear systems within teams to cope with such stresses – including having an environment that respects the identities of the members and encourages an open approach so that the issues can raised and discussed effectively. Resilience is not "possessed or not possessed" but "flows through the team in response to the situation it faces" [18]. The awareness and responsiveness of the team to these issues is crucial for the development of resilience so that the team creates an environment that allows for flexibility and responsiveness to adversity – whether from outside or within the team.

Support of Professionals Within a Team

Any professional involved in the care of a person with a neurological disease may face stress and distress. This may be due to conflict – with the patient, family, team members, other teams – or be related to the losses and stresses experienced by patients with progressive disease. There is a need to ensure that support systems are developed to help team members cope with these specific stressors, as well as the stresses that may occur within our own lives and relationships.

The care of people with progressive neurological disease, ultimately progressing to death, can be stressful for all involved – including the professional carers. This may be:

- Repeated again and again in some institutional settings and team (e.g., hospice)
- Rare for some teams, when death does occur, but this is rare within a small patient group

  However, in both situations, support may be helpful, and attention to the issues of stress – for individuals and within the team itself – needs to be considered.

Moreover, the stress experienced within a team may be:

- An individual reaction – every person reacting to stress differently – often with their own stresses within their own lives
- A team issue – where the whole team is affected
- Team conflict – when stresses affect the members differently, and this leads to issues within the team and between team members.

Team Stresses

Everyone experiences stresses differently, and there may be certain factors that affect the reactions and response to stressful circumstances:

- Age – younger caregivers report more stresses, manifest stress, and have fewer coping strategies [20]
- Gender – women seem to experience more strains within their roles and report suicidal ideation more often [21]. However, women also seem to report greater satisfaction with their job and greater well-being.
- Personality – people often develop ways to cope with the issues they face. There are both positive strategies – allowing expression of their feelings and issues – and negative, when issues are suppressed and not acknowledged but continue to have an effect on them.

In hospices, there is evidence that team members have greater self-awareness and a clearer personal philosophy –"buying into the present."

It has been suggested that "hardiness" – commitment, control, and challenge – is associated with decreased burnout and the sense of control in life, and the working environment may be helpful in enabling people to cope with stress at work.

- Spirituality and religious belief systems – there is evidence that a sense of spirituality may help caregivers find meaning in what they do, allowing a balance in life. In some circumstances, a sense of spirituality may encourage someone to undertake a commitment to service others and give real sense of meaning to both work and relationships.

Coping with Stressors

Within teams, there may be different ways of coping with the stresses of work and there may be stressors within the team itself

- Role overload – with increasing workload.
- Role conflict – with team members in conflict regarding both the work itself and ways of coping with the work and stressors.

- Team conflict – with communication issues within the team as described above.
- Issues of coping with dying and death – as the close connections with the patient and family can cause stress to all involved [18], and there may be issues with different team members finding the issues relating to being clear as to boundaries with patients and their families vary, causing conflict.
- Multiple loss – there may be issues of facing multiple losses when caring for people with progressive neurological disease – the patient themselves face multiple losses of mobility, speech, swallowing , and cognition – and team members are closely involved in these losses, and an accumulation of grief when patients die, which may lead to depression.

There is a need to ensure adequate time and commitment to consider the issues of stress and loss. These are often missed, and in the continual workload, the pressure on team members is minimized and not always appreciated, with long-term sequelae of team pressures, discord, and potentially burnout and illness. Within teams, there is the need to have clear opportunities for discussion and acceptance of these stresses. Team members may need help and continuing support. Clinical supervision may allow the issues to be recognized and addressed in a positive way. However, there are often personal issues that influence the reactions and abilities of people to cope with work and team pressures. The approach will be individual, accepting the interaction between the team and personal issues and stresses.

Every team member has a responsibility to find their personal strategies for coping with the stresses they face. Within teams, there is the need to ensure that these needs are recognized, time is allowed to express emotions and to debrief if necessary, clinical supervision allows opportunities for wider discussion and support, and all team members are aware of the needs of other members of the team so that there can be mutual support and growth.

Conclusion

The involvement of a wider team, with many different disciplines all adding their own knowledge and expertise to the person's care, can improve patient and family care. For a person with a progressive neurological disease, facing the end of their life, this approach is even more important.

The multidisciplinary approach will enable the correct assessment of the patient and family, leading all the team members providing their own expertise and care in an effective and coordinated approach. The aims and plan of care can be communicated to all concerned, and common goals can be agreed with other teams involved in the care. The complexity of care that may be required for a patient with neurological care may only be provided by this coordinated approach. Moreover, the team will also be able to support not only the patient and family but the team members themselves, when facing the stresses of coping progressive disease and potential conflict, and thus achieve higher satisfaction in their roles and continue to develop and improve the care they offer.

The multidisciplinary team approach will allow all aspects of the patient's needs and care to be considered and allow involvement of the most appropriate professional help at the most appropriate time for the patient and family. A highly performing team will enable the patient and family to maximize the care that can be provided and to live as full a life as possible.

References

1. Department of Health National service framework for long term conditions. 2005. http://www.dh.gov.uk/en/Publicationsandstatistics/Publications/PublicationsPolicyAndGuidance/DH_4105361
2. National Institute for Clinical Excellence. Improving supportive and palliative care in cancer. London: National Institute for Clinical Excellence; 2004.
3. Speck P. Team or group- spot the difference. In: Speck E, editor. Teamwork in palliative care: fulfilling or frustrating. Oxford: Oxford University Press; 2006.
4. Katzenbach JR, Smith DK. The wisdom of teams. Boston: Harvard Business School Press; 1992.
5. Haugen DF, Nauck F, Caraceni A. The core team and the extended team. In: Hanks G, Cherny NI, Christakis NA, Fallon M, Kaasa S, Portenoy RK, editors. Oxford textbook of palliative medicine. 4th ed. Oxford: Oxford University Press; 2010.
6. Drinka TJK. Interdisciplinary geriatric teams: approaches to conflict as indicators of potential to model teamwork. Educ Gerontol. 1994;20:87–103.
7. The National Collaborating Centre for Chronic Conditions. Parkinson's disease: national clinical guideline for diagnosis and management in primary and secondary care. London: Royal College of Physicians; 2006.
8. Kozlowski SWJ, Chao GT. Macrocognition, team learning and team knowledge: origins, emergence and measurement. In: Salas E, Fiore SM, Letsky MP, editors. Theories of team cognition: cross-disciplinary perspectives. Abingdon: Routledge; 2011.
9. Beckhard R. Optimising team building effectiveness. J Contemp Bus. 1972;1:23–32.
10. Carroll JM, Conventino G, Rosson MB, Ganoe CH. Towards a conceptual model of common ground in teamwork. In: Letsky MP, Warner NW, Fiore SM, Smith CAP (eds) Macrorecognition in teams; theories and methodologies. Aldershot: Ashgate Publishing; 2008. p. 87–106.
11. Freeman M, Miller C, Ross M. The impact of individual philosophies of teamwork on multi-professional practice and the implications for education. J Interprof Care. 2000;14:237–47.
12. Speck P. Maintaining a healthy team. In: Speck E, editor. Teamwork in palliative care: fulfilling or frustrating. Oxford: Oxford University Press; 2006.
13. Randall F, Downie RS. The philosophy of palliative care: critique and reconstruction. Oxford: Oxford University Press; 2006.
14. Ministry of Justice. Mental Capacity Act London 2005.
15. Royal College of Physicians/National Council for Palliative Care/British Society of Rehabilitation Medicine. Long term neurological conditions: management at the interface between neurology, rehabilitation and palliative care. Concise Guidance to Good Practice series, No 10. London; Royal College of Physicians, 2008.
16. Jeffrey D. Communication between professionals. In: Hanks G, Cherny NI, Christakis NA, Fallon M, Kaasa S, Portenoy RK, editors. Oxford textbook of palliative medicine. 4th ed. Oxford: Oxford University Press; 2010.
17. Department of Health. A vision for the future: report of the chief nursing officer. London: HMSO; 1993.
18. Payne M. Resilient multiprofessional teams. In: Monroe B, Oliviere D, editors. Resilience in palliative care – achievement in adversity. Oxford: Oxford University Press; 2007.

19. Fraser MW, Richman JM, Galinsky MJ. Risk, protection, and resilience: toward a conceptual framework for social science practice. Soc Work Res. 1999;23:129–208.
20. Vachon MLS. Occupational stress in the care of the critically ill, the dying and the bereaved. New York: Hemisphere Press; 1987.
21. Payne N. Occupational stressors and coping as determinants of burnout in female hospice nurses. J Adv Nurs. 2001;33:396–405.

Chapter 7
Advance Care Planning

Simon Chapman

Abstract People with progressive neurological disease face many challenges and changes in their condition – both physical and cognitive. Advance care planning allows the person to make their wishes known, while they are still able to do so. If they are not able to make decisions for themselves later in the disease progression, due to loss of communication or loss of capacity due to cognitive changes, those involved in their care can be aware of these wishes and plan care appropriately. In this way advance care planning allows clearer decision-making for all concerned – the person with the neurological condition, their family and carers, and the professionals involved in their care.

Keywords Capacity • Advance care planning • Decision-making • MCA • ADRT

Case Vignette

Albert Peters was a 66-year-old married man, who had been an engineer. After retirement, he became more breathless and felt unwell. A chest x-ray was normal, and he put all the changes down to "old age." When he developed pain in his knee, an arthroscopy was arranged. However, after the procedure, he did not start to breathe again and was transferred to the intensive care unit. He was found to be in respiratory failure and was unable to breathe by himself. A tracheotomy was performed, and he was dependent on a ventilator to keep him alive – when any activity was undertaken to clean the tube or adjust the machine, he became very breathless and distressed. During this period, a diagnosis of motor neuron disease was made.

S. Chapman
Director of Policy & Parliamentary Affairs,
The National Council for Palliative Care,
The Fitzpatrick Building, 188-194 York Way, London N7 9AS, UK
e-mail: s.chapman@ncpc.org.uk

D. Oliver (ed.), *End of Life Care in Neurological Disease*,
DOI 10.1007/978-0-85729-682-5_7, © Springer-Verlag London 2013

Following admission to the hospice, to plan discharge home, he talked openly of his poor prognosis and of dying. He had been in hospitals for several months and was determined to go home and stay at home. He made it clear that he would prefer to die at home than be readmitted to hospital. Before his discharge, hospice staff discussed with Albert and his wife what he wanted for the future. He was very clear that he did not want to be readmitted to hospital, nor receive cardiopulmonary resuscitation, or continued ventilation if his condition deteriorated, but instead wanted to remain at home and receive care to keep him comfortable. It was decided that he would complete an advance decision to refuse both CPR and ventilation. He realized that this could result in his death. He completed an advance decision, which was signed and witnessed, and complied with all the requirements of the Mental Capacity Act and was discharged to his home.

He enjoyed his time at home and was able to go out to see his grandson play football and his granddaughter dance in a show. His condition deteriorated one morning, and as he had wished, he was given an injection to relieve his distress and was not transferred to hospital and died at home later that day with his family with him.

His family were pleased that his wishes had been upheld and felt that the completion of the advance decision had allowed them all to discuss the issues

Introduction

As people living with neurological conditions approach the end of life, whether they die with or from their condition, it is important that the neurological condition is understood and managed appropriately. Many of those people will experience impaired cognition and ability to communicate, in addition to the physical impact of their condition. It will also be possible, in many instances, to anticipate the types of choice and decisions that might need to be made in respect of their daily living treatment and care as they approach and reach the end of life.

Embarking upon a process of advance care planning while the person retains capacity, so that they can discuss and document their preferences and choices about their future care, is therefore an essential step if they are to receive high-quality person-centered care that enables them to live and be cared for in the place of their choosing until the end of life. It is a vital part of delivering care based on the principle "nothing about me without me." Moreover, commitment to helping people plan their future care, whatever their future mental capacity, contributes significantly to enhancing their dignity.

Hence it is unsurprising that extending advance care planning so that it is offered to all people identified as approaching the end of life is seen as a core component in national and local strategies to develop end of life care [1].

Advance care planning is not only seen as good practice and an important policy tool to improve care but, in some countries, is supported by legislation. For example, in England and Wales, the Mental Capacity Act 2005 (the MCA) [2], contains provisions about:

- Assessment of capacity
- Supporting people so that they can make decisions for themselves where possible
- Best interests decision-making, if a person lacks capacity to make a decision themselves
- Advance decisions to refuse treatment
- Proxy decision-making through lasting power of attorney
- A duty to consult those close to the person lacking capacity when assessing their best interests

This importance of this legislative framework is that it lifts advance care planning beyond the realm of good practice to the sphere of rights, enforceability, and compliance. It protects both people who lack capacity to make a decision and those who then have to make a decision on their behalf. It means that if people decide to identify their preferences and choices, services and care providers have to respond; they cannot be ignored. Providers of health and social care have an obligation to ensure that their staff have been appropriately trained in communication and advance care planning, as part of ensuring legal compliance.

What Do We Mean by Advance Care Planning?

There are a number of important features about advance care planning.

- It is voluntary; people should not be forced to do it if they do not want to. While the benefits may seem obvious to professional carers, distress can be caused if people feel coerced into having a discussion they do not feel ready to have. It is therefore essential that, when advance care planning is offered to an individual, it is carried out by people with sufficient communication skills and training to be able to recognize the cues and signals being given and respond appropriately.
- People should be offered it at an appropriate moment so that they know it exists as a possibility. If they have wishes and preferences for their future care, and those have not been discussed and recorded, then, should they lose capacity in the future, it becomes much more unlikely they will get the care they would have wanted.
- Advance care planning is a process. People's attitudes and relationship with their condition changes over time. For example, at the time of receiving a diagnosis of multiple sclerosis, a person might be adamant that they would never want a PEG to be fitted. However, if that becomes necessary, in the great majority of cases, people give their consent for a PEG.

- It is important to keep under review what people have recorded about their wishes and preferences. The regularity of that review will depend on the individual's circumstances and the progression of the condition and should be decided accordingly.

The chief difference between advance care planning and care planning more generally is that advance care planning anticipates a future possible lack of capacity, whereas general care planning is what should happen for people with long-term conditions regardless of future capacity [4].

The chief purpose of advance care planning is to enable people to influence or control their future care. Many people with degenerative neurological conditions face the prospect that a time will come when they will no longer be able to make decisions about aspects of their lives, including some of the most important, personal, or intimate things that happen each day. This can be very daunting. The knowledge that it is possible to look ahead with your family and people close to you, as well as the health and care staff involved in your care, and record your wishes and preferences, and that what you have written down or said needs to be respected and taken into account, can be very reassuring. It can also prevent disagreement and distress arising in the future when decisions come to be made and the person lacks the capacity to decide themselves.

Box 7.1. Definition of Advance Care Planning

"Advance care planning is a voluntary process of discussion and review to help an individual who has capacity to anticipate how their condition may affect them in the future and, if they wish, set on record choices or decisions relating to their care and treatment so that these can then be referred to by their carers (whether professional or family carers) in the event that they lose capacity to decide once their illness progresses."

Capacity, care planning and advance care planning in life limiting illness: A Guide for Health and Social Care Staff

National End of Life Care Programme [3]

How Can People Use Advance Care Planning to Identify and Protect Their Wishes and Preferences?

The legal framework surrounding advance care planning does vary from country to country. This section will consider the impact of the MCA on advance care planning specifically in England and Wales.

The MCA [2] enables people to identify what they would like to happen in the future, should they lose capacity, and what they would not like to happen, with varying degrees of legal protection. There is in effect a menu or toolkit of different things they can do. They can

- Make advance statements about their wishes, preferences, and values
- Identify people they would like to be consulted about their best interests
- Identify people they would like not to be consulted

If they wish to go further than that, they can

- Make an advance decision to refuse specified treatments
- Appoint one or more people to make decisions for them, using a lasting power of attorney

Advance Statements

These statements can cover all manner of things about a person's wishes and preferences in relation to their care and treatment:

- Where they want to be cared for
- What food they like or dislike
- How they like to be washed
- Their preferred music
- Their spiritual beliefs, values
- Important relationships
- Any other aspect of care/values/areas of importance they would like to record

The information they contain will help inform people who have to make best interests decisions about the person in the event they lose the capacity to make a decision themselves. The MCA states that where a person lacks capacity to make a particular decision, any written statement of their wishes, preferences beliefs, and values must be taken into account by the person who makes the decision on their behalf [2].

It should be emphasized that the MCA does not say that an advance statement must always be followed. They must be considered and taken into account when assessing a person's best interests by the team involved in the person's care. Where there is a well-documented advance statement, efforts should be made to give effect to it, unless it is clear that the person's best interests require that a different course be followed – such as a change in circumstances that the person may not have envisaged.

A number of forms and documents ("tools") have been created to enable advance statements to be recorded on the basis of what people have said in advance care planning discussions, or which are available to people to complete themselves should they wish to. It would always be advisable to speak with a health or social care professional to seek information and advice before completing an advance statement about those aspects of life. One example of these tools is the Preferred Priorities of Care document [5]. However, people do not need to use those documents and can write down their wishes and preferences themselves if they want to.

For somebody with a degenerative neurological condition which will reduce their capacity to decide and communicate, creating an advance statement has the potential to make a real difference to their quality and experience of care. It can mean that those who care for them in the future have a detailed picture about who they are, their likes, dislikes, wishes, and preferences which can inform their future care. Knowing that somebody prefers being showered to being given a bath, likes the taste of marmite, listening to jazz, spending time being outside, wearing green clothes, and so on, or none of those things, can be immensely helpful and reassuring for all concerned.

Nominating Other People to Be Consulted

The MCA says that if somebody has nominated another person to be consulted about their best interests, the views of that person should be taken into account when making decisions. Although the act does not specify it, the reverse is also true: It is possible for somebody to identify somebody whose views they might not want to be taken into account.

It is important to remember that, in this situation, decision-making still rests with the health and social care professionals responsible for the person's care. The nominated person is there to be consulted about the person's best interests but is not the decision maker. If somebody wants to authorize another person to make decisions on their behalf, they need to give them a lasting power of attorney (see below).

Case Study

Jane has multiple sclerosis. She is very close to her neighbor, Fran, who she sees almost every day, and they know each other very well. She has had many conversations with Fran about every part of life, including her condition and how she feels about the future, now that her condition is deteriorating. Jane also has a daughter, Sue, who lives a long way away. They see each other occasionally but are not particularly close, and Jane feels that Sue does not really understand her wishes and preferences and has not come to terms with the possibility of her approaching death. Jane tells her care team that she would like them to talk to Fran if they have to make decisions, as she knows her best. She also tells Fran, who agrees that she would do this, and this is recorded as part of an advance statement about Jane's wishes and preferences.

When Sue is told about this, she is initially upset that Jane has nominated Fran to be asked about her best interests. However, she is reassured that decisions would still have to be made in Jane's best interests. Realizing that Jane saw this as being so important helped Sue start to talk with Jane more openly about the future and what each of them felt.

Advance Decisions to Refuse Treatment

People with neurological conditions may decide that they want to refuse specific treatments in the future. The MCA provides the framework for this. People can refuse any manner of treatment, for example, they may have found that a particular pressure bandage is uncomfortable. However, the decisions are very commonly those involved in the context of life-sustaining treatment.

There are a number of important differences between advance statements and advance decisions to refuse treatment (ADRT). Advance statements can cover any aspect of care and treatment, including requests, likes, and dislikes. An ADRT only covers refusals of specific treatments. So, a preference to be cared for at home as long as possible, coupled with a wish not to be readmitted to hospital, is an advance statement. However, a wish not to have cardiopulmonary resuscitation or ventilation is an advance decision to refuse treatment.

The most significant difference is that while advance statements have legal status, in that as a matter of law, they must be considered and taken into account, an ADRT that meets all the requirements of the MCA will be legally binding and must be followed.

Although an ADRT can apply in all circumstances, it may well be that people want them to apply in some circumstances but not others. For example, people might want to refuse antibiotics for a chest infection but not a urinary tract infection. If that is the case, care needs to be taken to specify the circumstances in which the refusal applies.

Case Study

Amir has a degenerative neurological condition which is deteriorating. He realizes that the end of his life is approaching. He has had several admissions to hospital for chest infections, which he has found increasingly stressful, and has decided that he now wants to live out the time remaining to him at home. He discusses this with his consultant and says that the next time he has a chest infection he would like to refuse antibiotics and remain at home. His consultant helps him complete an advance decision to refuse treatment that specifies that Amir is refusing antibiotics in the event that he has a chest infection. Amir also discusses these issues with his family and says that he wants now to stay at home. He records this in an advance care plan.

Amir's condition starts to worsen on a Friday night. His family calls the duty GP and asks her to help make Amir comfortable. The GP initially thinks that Amir should go to hospital. However, she reads the advance decision to refuse treatment and his statement saying that he wants to stay at home and agrees that his best interests would be to remain at home. She helps ensure that his symptoms are properly controlled so that he is comfortable. Amir dies 36 hours later at home with his family around him.

The ADRT only applies if the person does not have capacity to make the decision. If the person does have capacity, they should be asked whether or not they wish to consent to the treatment being offered. It is only if they do not have capacity to consent or refuse treatment that the ADRT should be referred to.

If somebody wants to refuse treatment that is or is potentially life-sustaining, the MCA requires that the ADRT must be written down, signed, witnessed, and contain a declaration that the decision applies even if the person's life is at risk as a result.

Lasting Powers of Attorney

As part of the advance care planning process, a person might decide that they would like to appoint somebody close to them to make decisions on their behalf. This can be done by giving somebody a lasting power of attorney (LPA). There are two kinds of LPA:

- One covering decisions about people's property and financial affairs.
- One covering their personal welfare, which would include their health and social care.

This is a bureaucratic process. LPAs must be filled out using a standard form from the Office of the Public Guardian [6]. They must be registered, and a fee is payable.

The holder (or "donee") of the LPA must make decisions about the person's care and treatment in their best interests. So, for example, they must take into account any advance statement the person has made.

Giving another person the authority to make decisions about your personal welfare, should you lose capacity is a significant responsibility. People giving LPAs should make sure that they trust the people they give them to. It would also be wise to ensure that an LPA is supported by a detailed advance statement, setting out people's wishes and preferences, to guide the donee of the LPA.

Mental Capacity

It should always be remembered that advance care planning and the different possible outcomes described above anticipate a time when a person lacks capacity to make particular decisions. However, the MCA makes it clear that there is a duty to support people so that, so far as is practicable, they can make their own decisions [2].

This is very important for people with neurological conditions. A 2012 court case involved a man with advanced MND who wanted to make an advance decision to refuse life-sustaining treatments. He communicated with his wife and health-care team using eye movements. The court ruled that he did have capacity to make an advance decision to refuse treatment and emphasized that total clarity was needed about what his wishes were [7]. Even though this man had very limited ability to communicate, with support he was still able to make his wishes known.

There is therefore an obligation to think carefully about what can be done to support people so that they can understand, weigh, and make judgements about information so as to make their decision and then to communicate it. Use of simple language, writing things down, giving them time and space in which to reflect are all important. The advice and support of a speech and language therapist may be helpful in facilitating communication. Wherever possible, people's autonomy should be supported and respected, so they can make their own decisions.

It should also be remembered that capacity is decision-specific. A person might be able, with support, to be able to make decisions about what they want to wear, or how they want to spend the day, but be unable to make more complex decisions, such as about their finances or their medical treatment. People should not be regarded as having a "blanket" capacity, covering all decisions and even when somebody might not have capacity to make a specific decision, the MCA states that as good practice they should still be involved, as they might have insights to contribute to the decision-maker.

Language

Using jargon-free language is an important aspect of supporting people. Many people find even the language of "advance care planning" quite off-putting. Language such as "planning for the future" or "making sure we know what you'd like if you become unable to decide yourself" can be more accessible. There is a tendency to use jargon and acronyms in all systems and health and social care is no exception. Care must be taken to ensure that language is used to explore concepts and record wishes that is appropriate and understood by the individual concerned.

Conclusion

Advance care planning is intended to benefit people who face impaired capacity, and those close to them, to help them plan and influence their future care. Careful discussion with people with neurological disease, their families, and their carers can allow their wishes to be known and then recorded. This may then allow their care to be the most appropriate for their specific needs and wishes, even if they cannot express their wishes at the time.

Further Resources

A great deal has been written about advance care planning, end of life decision-making, and the Mental Capacity Act. Useful publications include:

- Planning for Your Future Care (2012). National End of Life Care Programme
- The Mental Capacity Act in Practice: Guidance for End of Life Care (2008). The National Council for Palliative Care
- Treatment and care toward the end of life: good practice in decision making (2010). The General Medical Council
- Decisions relating to cardiopulmonary resuscitation (2007). The resuscitation Council, the British Medical Association, and the Royal College of Nursing

Useful websites include:

- The Dying Matters coalition – on opening up discussions about the end of life www.dyingmatters.org
- The National End of Life Care Programme www.endoflifecareforadults.nhs.uk
- The National Council for Palliative Care www.ncpc.org.uk
- The Office of the Public Guardian www.justice.gov.uk/about/opg

References

1. Department of Health. End of Life Care Strategy – promoting high quality care for all adults at the end of life. Department of Health. London. 2008.
2. Department of Justice. Mental Capacity Act. Department of Justice. London. 2005. http://www.justice.gov.uk/protecting-the-vulnerable/mental-capacity-act. Accessed 5.5.12.
3. National End of Life Care Programme. Capacity, care planning and advance care planning in life limiting illness: a Guide for Health and Social Care Staff. London: National End of Life Care Programme; 2011.
4. National End of Life Care Programme. The differences between general care planning and decisions made in advance. London: National End of Life Care Programme, 2010. http://www.endoflifecareforadults.nhs.uk/publications/differencesacpadrt. Accessed 5.5.12.
5. National Preferred Priorities of Care review Team. Preferred Priorities of Care National End of Life Care Programme. London. 2007. http://www.endoflifecareforadults.nhs.uk/tools/core-tools/preferredprioritiesforcare. Accessed 5.5.12.
6. Department of Justice. http://www.justice.gov.uk/forms/opg. Accessed 5.5.12.
7. Reported in the Daily Telegraph newspaper 1 May 2012. http://www.telegraph.co.uk/health/healthnews/9239559/Living-wills-need-to-be-completely-clear-rules-judge.html.

Chapter 8
Care at the End of Life

Nigel P. Sykes

Abstract Good end of life care always requires preparation, but this is especially so in neurological disease, where the signs of impending death can be unclear and there may be a substantial period of mental incapacity. A sensitive process of advance care planning can enable both patient and family to face what lies ahead and makes choices about what style of care would be preferred. It also facilitates both psychological and spiritual preparedness and also an awareness of what symptoms are likely to occur and how they can be managed. Achieving all this needs cooperation and mutual learning between neurology, palliative care, and rehabilitation, in addition to support for long-term care staff who may be involved. Symptoms, which will center around issues of breathing, restlessness, hydration, and pain, have to be anticipated and appropriate drugs made available for their management. Ventilation, whether noninvasive or via tracheostomy, deserves careful consideration with respect both to starting it and to when and how it may be withdrawn. The importance of good care at the end of life cannot be overestimated, as this phase of the illness leaves a powerful impression in the minds of those who were close to the patient and is influential in shaping their attitudes both to illness and to healthcare.

Keywords Neurology • Palliative care • Terminal care • Advance care planning Symptom control • Carers • Team support

Case History

Jack was a 75-year-old man with a 2-year history of limb onset motor neuron disease. By the time he was admitted to a hospice to give his family a period of respite, he needed assistance to stand and was beginning to have problems with swallowing. The community palliative care team had initiated discussion

N.P. Sykes, M.A., FRCP, FRCGP
St. Christopher's Hospice, Lawrie Park Road,
London SE26 6DZ, UK
e-mail: n.sykes@stchristophers.org.uk

D. Oliver (ed.), *End of Life Care in Neurological Disease*,
DOI 10.1007/978-0-85729-682-5_8, © Springer-Verlag London 2013

with him about the possible benefit of having a gastrostomy tube inserted, but Jack had consistently made it clear that he did not want this intervention. Although not particularly breathless at the level of physical activity his strength allowed, Jack had begun to have more difficulty in sleeping and sometimes complained of headache in the mornings. The caring team had suggested a respiratory function assessment at the local hospital, but Jack had continued to be reluctant to undergo this as he wanted to remain at home and did not want his life extended.

The admission was prolonged because Jack and his family decided that continued care at home was now too difficult, and so a nursing home placement was sought. Over this time, his swallowing was deteriorating, although he remained able to take thickened fluids without evidence of aspiration. He was noted to have reduced chest expansion, but this had not apparently altered during his stay.

On the day of his death, he was noted to be generally less well on waking in the morning, complaining of widespread discomfort throughout his body and intermittent breathlessness. It was agreed with him that nursing home transfer, which had been imminent, should be deferred. Jack accepted administration of medication subcutaneously via a syringe driver, and this was set up at midday with morphine sulfate 7.5 mg/24 h combined with glycopyrronium bromide 1.2 mg/24 h. His speech became less distinct during the course of the day, but he remained able to make himself understood by expressions if not always by words.

That evening Jack settled to sleep at his usual time. At 4.30 the next morning, he was noted by nursing staff to be peaceful, but respiration was shallow. Five minutes later Jack's breathing ceased.

Comment: Although there was a background of gradual deterioration in Jack's MND, the changes that culminated in his death took place within about 24 h. In particular, his respiratory function declined sharply and, as is characteristic in this condition, he died from respiratory failure. The amount of medication required for his comfort was small. It was recognized by staff that the changes in his condition heralded death within a short while, and it was possible to warn his family of what lay ahead. Jack himself had consistently been clear that he wanted no life-prolonging interventions and in the course of his last day sought reassurance that the caring team's aim was simply to maximize his comfort and not to extend his life.

Introduction

For the sake of argument, "end of life" will be defined here as the part of the illness course that contains the final deterioration that culminates in death. This is the time when specialist palliative care, if available, is most likely to be needed in order to meet the challenges of the patient's symptoms and the distress of those around them. Both will be much less, though, if this phase of care can be built on a foundation of competent palliation extending back over the prior course of the condition. Therefore, it should not be supposed that what will be described here contains all that good palliative care is about, or that a person who receives such attention only as their life is drawing to a close has thereby received adequate palliation of their disease.

A principal difficulty in delivering end of life care in neurological disease is the recognition of when this phase has been reached. In diseases such as Parkinson's disease (PD) and multiple sclerosis (MS) that extend over many years and in which death results primarily through respiratory or other infection, marked debility, including cognitive dysfunction, may be present for a prolonged period and does not necessarily herald death – see Chap. 2. Even in motor neuron disease (MND) the extent of nonrespiratory disability is not necessarily a reliable guide to prognosis, especially in younger people, but it is claimed that the requirement for physical aids and adaptations marks approximately the halfway point of the disease career, with gastrostomy feeding at about 80 % and ventilatory support at 80–90 % [1].

However, the terminal phase can be short, even sudden, in MND and conditions such as progressive supranuclear palsy (PSP) or multisystem atrophy (MSA), in which the predominant mechanism of death is respiratory failure. In a series of 124 MND patients cared for until death, 40 % deteriorated suddenly and died within 12 h; a further 18 % had died within 24 h of a change in condition first being noticed [2]. In MSA, there is estimated to be around a one in five chance of sudden death. On the one hand, therefore, there is a risk that a patient's family may experience a number of false alarms, when a deterioration heralded as fatal proves not be so after all, and there is ongoing prognostic uncertainty. On the other, they experience what seems a catastrophically sudden demise as death occurred before they had been prepared to expect it. In either case, the key support for both patient and family is anticipatory preparation by the caring team, working with them to enable a process of advance care planning and also to make sure that adequate services, equipment, and medications are available ahead of any end of life crisis arising.

Where respiratory failure is the prime cause of death, end of life care can be altered completely by the use of assisted ventilation in the presence of gastrostomy feeding. It has become clear that noninvasive ventilation (NIV) can extend life significantly [3], but eventually respiratory failure occurs despite it. When this happens, medication will be needed for breathlessness in the same way as when NIV has not been used, and the ventilator may then be withdrawn. The alternative is to make a transition to tracheostomy ventilation, which can extend life indefinitely to the extent that functional deterioration continues to the point of a locked-in state. The timing and nature of the terminal event are then the result of the availability of assisted ventilation within the prevailing health-care system, whether tracheostomy ventilation is offered to a patient whose NIV is ceasing to be adequate and whether it is decided to withdraw tracheostomy ventilation at some point in the patient's disease progression.

Patient and Family Support

The key means of supporting both patients facing life-shortening illness and their family has in recent years increasingly been seen to be a process of advance care planning. By this is meant an opportunity, which may be spread over several conversations and quite a long period, for the person who is ill to learn what they wish to know about their condition and to express their preferences about how they wish to be looked after, where and by whom. Advance care planning has the purpose of improving health-care outcomes by making sure that decision making is shared between patients and professionals. It also enables clinical care to continue to accord with a patient's informed decisions and preferences at a time when independent decisions are no longer possible, something that is particularly relevant to neurological diseases in view of the communication and cognitive difficulties that often arise in their later stages.

This is important not only for patients, who can feel that their personal views are known and will be respected, and clinicians, but also for families, who can be relieved of the burden of feeling that they have to make potentially weighty decisions on behalf of the patient without guidance. At the same time, the process can uncover disparities in hopes and expectations between patient and family that then have a chance of being resolved before they cause acrimony or practical difficulty.

It is helpful if the results of the advance care planning process are set down in writing and made accessible to others who are involved, both professionals and family or friends as appropriate. However, the dialogue may be sound or video recorded instead, or its outcomes put down in the health record. In England, this is known as a "statement of wishes and preferences" that, although not legally binding, has been promoted as a valuable tool to guide and improve end of life care [4]. However, with recognition by legal frameworks such as the Mental Capacity Act 2005 in England and the Patient Self-Determination Act 1991 in the USA, advance care planning can result in more binding outcomes in the form of either an instructional directive, otherwise known as a "living will" or an "advance decision to refuse treatment," or through the appointment of a person as proxy or attorney who is empowered to make decisions about medical treatment on behalf of the patient should they lose the capacity to decide these matters for themselves.

Advance decisions (or directives) originated as an attempt to oblige doctors to take notice of patients' desires regarding investigation and treatment. Since they cannot legally demand treatments but only refuse them, they have also been regarded as a way of reducing medical costs [5]. A number of advance decision templates have been produced, some of them disease specific, for example, for MND. Yet in general the uptake of this form of communication has been low, with evidence that it is most often adopted by the better educated and the better off [6]. A major limitation to the practical usefulness of advance decisions is that they are unenforceable if the situation they describe cannot clearly be recognized as the one that has actually arisen, either through the description being too vague or too specific. Although advance directives are a way of a patient ensuring that specific interventions such as ventilation or a gastrostomy placement are not performed on them, in general the evidence is that these documents have limited influence on doctors feeling that they know a patient's wishes or on the completion of Do Not Attempt Resuscitation orders. This is because the implementation of advance directives has not in general been accompanied by additional training in communication skills, and it is the emphasis on advance care planning as a process of communication that is a chief contributor to its value – see Chap. 7.

The unpressured process of advance care planning required if end of life care is going to go as well as possible both for patient and family needs the clinicians involved to recognize well ahead of time the eventual outcome of the disease, before it becomes too late to uncover and allay wishes and fears about the dying process and about where and how it should be handled. While the conversation has to go at the patient's pace and be directed by their concerns, it is vital that the professionals give them the opportunity to be aware of, and to explore, key options that may become available, such as gastrostomy insertion or noninvasive ventilation. These topics will arise out of conversations about the likely progression of the neurological symptoms, conversations that over time can lead naturally to a consideration of the end of life, what it will be like and how it can be handled. People vary in how much they are able to participate in such conversations and how fast the dialogue can go (which also depends on the rate of deterioration of the particular condition). But the other important variable is the skill of the professional in terms of their ability to communicate clearly and empathetically, their knowledge of the illness, and their personal readiness to converse about issues of mortality that may resonate for them personally. Without these types of skill, the ability of staff to help patients prepare for the end of their life will be compromised.

What topic areas might come into conversations preparing for end of life? Perhaps the principal ones are the following:

- Where will the patient be looked after and (not necessarily the same) where will they die?
- If the patient wants to be at home, what will be required of the family and what outside help can they get?
- Discussion of the sense of loss felt by both patient and family
- What to expect in terms of symptoms and changes in the patient's body?
- What can be done to relieve symptoms, in particular any symptoms associated with dying itself?

Place of Care and Death

Most terminally ill people want to be cared for in their own home. As the illness progresses and life becomes more difficult, the proportion wishing to stay at home reduces but still remains about 50 % [7]. Despite assistance from community nursing services that may be available, the brunt of home care is borne by the family.

Respite admissions to a hospice, hospital, or care home can help caregivers to recuperate and resume their task, or additional respite nursing help may be available for limited periods. However, for a significant number of families, there comes a point when they feel they can no longer look after the patient at home. For some families, it is important that their relative does not die in their home, even if they have been looked after there throughout the illness, because of the memories that would leave for the future. The patient himself may share the family perception, or there may be divergence, as there may be between different family members.

This is why there need to be conversations with patient and family about the preferred place of death if at all possible so that in case of a difference, there can be discussion and understanding, if not always agreement. Even if all are in agreement that admission is needed, family members may still be left with a sense of failure and of guilt that they have let their relative down. This might be especially marked if the ill person dies soon after admission, leading to feelings that "if only we had kept going that little bit longer we could have looked after him to the end." How well bereaved people cope with their loss is significantly affected by their memories of the events that led up to it, and it is important for their response in bereavement that families receive reassurance about the quality of their caring efforts prior to the admission and the appropriateness of seeking inpatient care now. It is also important that there are the facilities and encouragement to enable them to remain with the patient as death approaches, if that would be helpful to them. It is worth pointing out that even when death does take place in an inpatient setting, usually at least 80 % of the patient's last year of life will have been spent at home, and afterward the perception of families is that they have indeed cared for the person themselves [7].

Care of the Dying Person

Looking after a dying person is an experience few family members will be familiar with, and it can be both fatiguing and frightening. Effective professional support can make all the difference both to the quality of care that the patient receives and to the ability of informal carers to cope. Symptoms such as paralysis, loss of speech, and cognitive impairment that, to varying degrees, are often associated with progressive neurological diseases produce a feeling of impotence in all who care for people with them. This sensation, which can be uncomfortable even for knowledgeable professionals, may be disabling and extremely distressing for family caregiver and friends.

Without guidance as to what to expect as swallowing and respiration deteriorate, and how they can gain urgent help in a crisis, an episode of choking or breathlessness can be terrifying not only to patient but also to family. This also, of course, entails such help actually being available, which remains a challenge to health services in many regions. Crises do not occur tidily during ordinary working hours, and advice by telephone, even by video link, is not always an effective substitute for a face-to-face visit from a knowledgeable professional. Both patients and families have to be able to trust the help that is on offer, which places a responsibility on professionals to communicate accurately what that help is and then to deliver it when required. This is particularly difficult with less common neurological conditions that community health-care workers seldom see and hence frequently feel insecure to manage. An adequate palliative care service for such patients and those close to them therefore requires access to round-the-clock practical support in the home but also availability of round-the-clock advice for the professionals who deliver that support from others who are familiar with management of the late stages of these conditions.

Recognition of the Dying Phase

Although progressive functional deterioration is clear to everyone, family members may not recognize how this links with shortening of the prognosis. In gradually progressive conditions like PD or many cases of MS, it may be very difficult to judge life expectancy with any accuracy, but in a condition marked by respiratory impairment like MND where death can occur with little warning, this uncertainty is a feature that families deserve to be prepared for. Some professionals find it very difficult to be asked by patients for an estimate of prognosis, not only because any attempt at accuracy is likely to be misplaced but also because they fear that the answer will cause the person to give up. Relatives are even more likely to take this view. However, it can be a consolation to someone greatly disabled by their disease to be told that their condition will not go on for much longer. Naturally, an exact prognosis is impossible to judge and if a time is asked for the answer has to be relatively imprecise. Yet simply to be told that time appears short is not enough without an assurance of continued support and symptom control, because there is also the issue of ongoing hope.

There is evidence that the grounds for hope can change as illness progresses [8]. By the nature of neurological conditions, the basis of hope is not achievement of a cure. Instead there are likely to be initial hopes that the disease may be slower in its progression or relatively limited in its scope or that it may be contained by a therapeutic intervention. With the open but sensitive communication that is fundamental to effective advance care planning, the basis of hope can evolve as symptoms continue to develop to the relief of discomfort and for a peaceful end to life. For this change to occur, there needs to be a quality of communication and relationship not only between the caring team and the ill person but also with the patient's family, whose own emotional adjustment to the patient's condition will have a profound effect on the patient's quality of life and, indeed, quality of death.

Quality of life can be thought of as resulting from the degree of agreement between hopes and expectations on the one hand and the reality of their achievement on the other [9]. If there is a serious mismatch between activities a person regards as their principal source of satisfaction and their actual ability to pursue those activities, the results are frustration and a sense of meaninglessness. Caregivers have to work to help the patient to adjust their horizons and focus to achieve enjoyment and a sense of worth from activities that may be new or may previously have been discounted but which still lie within their capacity. This type of support is a major contribution of hospice day units. Naturally, the range of these activities becomes increasingly limited over time, but this aspect of care remains important right up to the onset of the terminal phase of the illness. It answers not only to the psychological needs of the individual but also the social and probably the spiritual as well.

Spiritual Care

By "spiritual" is meant the need to find within present existence a sense of meaning. How to define this is a matter for each person. It may, but often does not, involve a framework of religion and the idea of a God with whom it is possible to have a relationship. When religion is an important feature, the clerical involvement might be appropriate, but caregivers also have to be ready for a person to prefer to talk to them as someone who is not an official representative of religion and is unlikely to have all the answers. This can be challenging for staff, but it is an important task, as there is evidence that failure to meet spiritual needs – in the sense of a satisfactory achievement of meaning and purpose in life – is strongly linked with anxiety and depression in patients with advanced illness [10].

Symptom Management

When the end of life is considered, worries can arise because of fears that death will occur through suffocation or choking, or dominated by pain. None of these scenarios should occur in reality, and a family's need for accurate information on this point is at least as great as that of the patient. Attention to detail is important in symptom control so that by the time end of life care dawns, a capacity for competent symptom control should have been demonstrated and maintained. There is much in neurological disease that cannot be fully alleviated, but patients and families usually accept that there are limits to what medicine can achieve as long as the health-care team shows a commitment to stay alongside them and keep trying. Whatever the problems earlier on, it should be possible for the promise to be made that at the end distress can be controlled and that death need be neither painful nor frightening. Provided that the correct drugs are available and are administered in the right doses and combinations, the promise can be fulfilled [2, 11]; see page x.

Most bereaved people do not need specific bereavement care: they will work through the feelings of loss that are at sometime part of every individual's experience by themselves with the support of their own network of family and friends. For a minority, perhaps up to 25 %, their adjustment can be helped by specialist bereavement support, although this, unfortunately, is only unevenly available.

Team Support

Professionals caring for people with neurological conditions, particularly those working in a care home setting, may have known a patient over many years and grown close to them. For most such carers, the death of one of their patients is only an occasional event, and so they are unfamiliar both with picking up the onset of dying and also with the management of the symptoms of dying itself. There is an urgent need here to improve skills and confidence in end of life care and care planning that goes far beyond looking after people with neurological disease. Supportive programs employing two end of life care tools – an adapted version of the Gold Standards Framework [12] and the Liverpool Care Pathway for the Dying [13] – have shown promise of improving both care home staff confidence and practical outcomes for patients and families [14]. The value of such initiatives is not only the benefit that patients may derive from them but also the enhancement of morale they can provide for the caring team.

At the same time, it is important that when problems arise, there is accessible nursing and advice about palliative care. However, a key issue in the end of life care of people with progressive neurological conditions is that the teams who specialize in neurology or rehabilitation have the major involvement over the course of the illness but do not generally regard the management of dying as part of their remit and, being almost exclusively hospital-based, tend to lose sight of these patients once they are unable to make their way to clinic. Conversely, the palliative care specialists who are comfortable with looking after dying patients usually have their majority engagement with cancer and can feel uncertain with neurological diseases [15]. The situation is worsened by the relative rarity of some conditions, rendering it difficult to gain and maintain confidence in caring for affected patients. General practitioners, for whom end of life neurological care is even rarer, may feel yet more out of their depth. There is therefore much scope for better integration and the extension of joint working between specialists in neurology, palliative care, and neurorehabilitation in order to facilitate the exchange of expertise and ensure that the right skills are available for changing needs as they arise, with some existing examples of good practice [16].

The inevitable losses in functional ability arising over a longer or shorter period of time from neurological disease can cause a sense of impotence and frustration in caring staff as well as in patients. To a degree, these tensions are eased in the terminal phase, as the end comes into sight and the situation comes to resemble more closely that of people dying of cancer and other conditions. However, after the death, staff memories of care may be colored by feelings which derive from earlier stages of the illness. Together with the possibility that they will have known a neurological patient for a relatively long time, this risks leaving a residue of distress which might impair their ability to look after people with a similar condition in the future.

Hence as well as the availability of education covering the management of neurological palliation, it can be useful after the death for staff to meet together as a multiprofessional group to share of views about the care of a particular patient went. The discussion may identify ways in which care could be improved in the future, but it should also be a chance for congratulation on the things that went well. It should be a managerial responsibility to identify staff members who have particular problems resulting from the experience of care and, without imparting a sense of inadequacy, enable them to talk through the important issues confidentially either within the organization or with an independent counselor.

Management of Symptoms

Good symptom control at the end of life requires preparedness. It is a completely inadequate response to the onset of a distressing symptom if management has to wait for a doctor's order or the pharmacist's acquisition of the medication required. When the signs of the onset of dying are clear, and particularly as respiratory capacity shows serious reduction, a stock of key drugs should be made available on the ward or in the home ready for use. The categories of drug needed to cover most eventualities at the end of life are the following:

- Opioids
- Sedatives
- Anticholinergic agents

If the drugs are to be used at home, family members may be willing to administer them in a crisis if the buccal or, particularly, the gastrostomy route is available. Whether or not the family is willing to assume this responsibility following adequate guidance, locally agreed paperwork must be filled out to enable community nurses to give the drugs when needed.

A care pathway approach to the management of dying has been developed and is increasingly used in UK hospitals, hospices, and nursing homes [13]. Although primarily designed for the care of people with cancer, it is also relevant to those dying from neurological conditions.

The principal symptom issues that are likely to need attention at the end of life are inability to eat and drink, respiratory problems, pain, and restlessness or agitation.

Hydration and Nutrition

Ceasing to eat and then to drink is a normal accompaniment of the dying process, whatever the disease. However, these changes can be interpreted by people close to the patient as the cause rather than the result of the deterioration and so can give rise to much distress. This distinction needs to be sensitively discussed by the health-care staff involved, as the physiological or symptom-relieving role of artificial hydration at this stage is unclear [17], and it may exacerbate peripheral edema and respiratory secretions. Many people with advanced neurological disease have already had insertion of a gastrostomy tube because of the development of dysphagia, but in any progressive disease, the ability of the body to benefit from nutrition diminishes so that, in the absence of any survival or life quality benefit, it is usually appropriate to reduce the volume of feed or even stop it as the onset of dying is recognized [18].

Respiratory Symptoms

Respiratory Secretions

If bulbar weakness is present, retention of secretions in the upper airways can be a frequent problem long before the terminal phase. Even in the absence of specific bulbar deficits, any severely ill patient with reduced ability to cough can accumulate secretions in the upper airways, resulting in noisy breathing which if not always a distress to him may be so to carers. At the end of life, this problem is one that is best anticipated, as it is not easy to get rid of secretions which have already gathered. But if there is persistent chest infection, there are likely also to be purulent exudates present which cannot be prevented so that it is not possible to stop noisy breathing altogether. Hence the first step in management is to explain to the patient's family the mechanism of the noisy breathing, what is being done and what its limitations are, and reassure them that by this stage of their illness, the dying person is unlikely to be nearly as aware of the sounds as they are themselves.

Retained secretions are managed by the use of suction and anticholinergic drugs. Suction is not the mainstay of such management because, unless used carefully, it can damage the buccal mucosa, increase irritation and secretions, and cause distress as a result of pain, coughing, or gagging. Anticholinergic drugs reduce oral and airway secretions, increase bronchodilation, and inhibit spasm. These agents are said to relieve noisy breathing due to retained secretions at the end of life in 30–50 % of cases, but the lack of standardized measures and adequately designed studies means that reliable figures are not available [19]. However, the absence of better alternatives means that anticholinergics continue to be used probably more than their efficacy can really justify.

If an anticholinergic agent is already being given by gastrostomy, it can be continued and the dose increased if secretion retention is worsening. Atropine tends to be arousing, though, and should dose titration be required, it would at this stage be more appropriate to change to a more neutral drug, such as hyoscine butylbromide or glycopyrronium bromide. Hyoscine hydrobromide can also be used: although this is normally sedating, it can occasionally cause paradoxical arousal, but it does have the potential advantage of being available as a transdermal patch. These drugs should be started at the first sign of noisy breathing as no drug can dry up secretions that are already present. Any of these drugs can be given subcutaneously by syringe driver in combination with morphine and midazolam or levomepromazine.

Dose ranges are:

- Hyoscine butylbromide: 20 mg stat s.c.; 60–240 mg/24 h by s.c. infusion*
- Glycopyrronium bromide: 200–400 µg stat s.c.; 600 µg–1.2 mg/24 h by s.c. infusion
- Hyoscine hydrobromide: 400–800 µg stat s.c.; 1.2–2.4 mg/24 h by s.c. infusion

*Hyoscine butylbromide and glycopyrronium bromide are available as oral formulations. If required any of the three drugs can be given in their injectable form via a gastrostomy, but none has a license for this use or for use in a subcutaneous infusion using a syringe driver – this is in common with many drugs used in palliative care. All are very poorly absorbed enterally, and the effective dose may be tenfold higher than when the drug is administered subcutaneously.

Choking and Aspiration

If there is bulbar impairment, the resulting dysphagia gives rise to choking sensations caused by food particles or thick secretions lodging in the upper airway. These feelings are both uncomfortable and frightening with patients fearing that will choke to death, especially as choking becomes more frequent as the disease progresses. In fact, there is evidence that death does not occur in this way [2, 11], and both patients and families need a clear message that choking episodes are alarming but not fatal. Aspiration of secretions are likely to contribute to the chest infection that is almost universal in those who die after an identifiable terminal phase and that probably often contributes to noisy breathing at the end of life. If, despite attempts to resolve the secretions, the breathing appears to be a source of distress at the very end of life, the most appropriate and effective response is to lessen the awareness of it by use of opioids and sedatives as discussed below.

Breathlessness

In any terminal illness, regardless of the involvement of the chest, breathlessness appears to increase as death approaches. It cannot be removed in the way that pain often can, but it should be possible to provide a significant degree of relief. Among neurological conditions, it is those that cause increasing respiratory weakness, such as MND, PSP, MSA, or Duchenne's muscular dystrophy (DMD), that are particularly prone to cause breathlessness at the close of life. This situation can be completely altered by the use of tracheostomy ventilation (TV) or NIV. In the case of NIV, the hours of use tend gradually to increase until it is being used continuously, or almost so. Ultimately, it becomes insufficient in the face of worsening respiratory weakness until either TV is instituted or a respiratory crisis occurs.

TV, on the other hand, can maintain life indefinitely to the point of the patient becoming "locked in" with no effective means of communication. This raises difficult ethical issues, especially if ventilation was started in an emergency without prior consultation with the patient, as has been reported in up to 25 % of cases of its use. Adequate palliative care and appropriate anticipatory planning should prevent such situations arising, but when they have the patient is faced with a decline from which there is no foreseeable natural exit and their family with major impacts upon their lives and, possibly, finances. There then needs to be consideration of a process of ventilator withdrawal, which is inevitably emotionally fraught for all concerned but which, with careful preparation, can even be achieved in the home setting [20].

Oxygen is not an appropriate therapy for the palliation of breathlessness unless hypoxia is demonstrated. Many breathless terminally ill people are not hypoxic, and the apparatus surrounding oxygen administration is an unnecessary encumbrance. If a patient is hypercapnic, and retaining carbon dioxide as a result of respiratory failure, the stimulus for breathing may be hypoxia, and additional oxygen may depress respiratory drive and increase respiratory failure or even cause death. Opioids and benzodiazepines are the principal drugs used for this purpose. Both oral and parenteral opioids can reduce breathlessness without precipitating respiratory depression [21]. Nebulized opioids have not been shown to be effective. Although initially often used on an as required basis, opioids are also used regularly for this indication and can be given by subcutaneous infusion. The dose used depends on that previously used for pain (if any) and is titrated against response.

There is less evidence for the use of benzodiazepines for breathlessness [22], but anxiety is often both a result of, and a contributor to, dyspnea, and so the use of this group of drugs as anxiolytics and muscle relaxants is logical. Lorazepam is rapidly effective for anxiety and breathlessness by the sublingual route, although controlled trial evidence is lacking. Midazolam, usually given subcutaneously but, in a crisis, occasionally buccally and rarely intravenously, is also frequently used in the palliative care management of breathlessness. Small initial doses of 1.25–2.5 mg can be titrated against response, and midazolam can be combined for subcutaneous infusion with morphine and other opioids, whose action it complements.

A phenothiazine can be used instead of the benzodiazepine, for example, chlorpromazine or the more sedating levomepromazine. Both have an antiemetic effect, if this is important, and there is limited evidence that chlorpromazine can palliate breathlessness [23]. Watch should be kept for myoclonic jerking, but the lowering of the fit threshold that these drugs induce is not a problem in end of life care in MND. Levomepromazine can be given by subcutaneous infusion and combined with opioids or midazolam, but chlorpromazine causes too many skin reactions to be given by this route.

Relief of breathlessness is one of the very few cases in which symptom control may sometimes shorten life. The objective in relieving breathlessness is to reduce awareness of breathing but not respiratory drive, a balance that in practice can be difficult to achieve. Ethically, the attempt to make a distressed patient more comfortable is defensible as long as causing death was not the doctor's intended method of achieving this outcome [24]. It should be made clear to the patient's family and friends how critically ill he is and how, as a result, efforts to ease severe breathlessness might further reduce his already brief life expectancy.

Restlessness and Agitation

Some degree of confusion has been reported in at least 80 % of dying people and can give rise to restlessness or even agitation. These unfocused motor disturbances need to be distinguished from myoclonus, which is a coordinated, sporadic contraction of particular muscle groups. Myoclonus can occur in clear consciousness and may be due to drugs, notably opioids and phenothiazines. Its appearance near the end of life may indicate increasing plasma drug levels as a result of deteriorating renal function.

Restlessness usually occurs in reduced consciousness, which is almost universal for a shorter or longer period in deaths from progressive diseases. In addition, mental impairment is common in advanced MS, PD, and PSP and is increasingly recognized in MND. Whether or not restlessness and agitation represent distress, they appear to carers to do so. The first step in management is to check for reversible exacerbating factors such as urinary retention, fecal loading, or hypoxia. A patient unable to smoke may experience nicotine withdrawal, the symptoms of which may benefit from a transdermal nicotine patch. Although it has been claimed that the incidence of delirium can be reduced by maintaining hydration and changing the opioid where this type of drug is being used, this has proved hard to replicate, and the value of additional fluid at the end of life is uncertain [17].

Although restlessness and agitated delirium are the most commonly cited indications for sedative use in palliative care, it is important that this is not the only response. Reversible factors have been mentioned, and some patients appear to settle if they sense the presence of someone sitting by their side. Not everyone at the end of life can receive such reassurance, however, and in this situation, the only practicable means of relieving distress is the use of sedatives. The aim of sedative use is *not* to induce sleep but to ease the signs of distress. Just as morphine doses are titrated toward against the pain response, so the sedative dose is titrated until distress is relieved [25]. When adequate relief has been obtained, no further dose increase is made. The use of sedatives in this way is not associated with shortening of life [26]. Communication both with relatives and between members of the caring team is important before and during sedative use so that the aims of treatment are understood by all.

The most commonly used drug for palliation of restlessness and agitation is the benzodiazepine midazolam, although diazepam can also be used as rectal suppositories or as liquid via a gastrostomy, given as required or twice or three times a day.

Table 8.1 Conversion ratios from oral opioids to subcutaneous morphine

Oral opioid	To obtain dose of s.c. morphine divide by:
Morphine	2
Tramadol	8
Codeine	16
Oxycodone	1
Hydromorphone	Multiply by 4

Midazolam is given subcutaneously and combines satisfactorily with opioid and anticholinergic agents in a syringe driver: an initial dose is 2.5 mg as a single injection or 10 mg/24 h by a continuous subcutaneous infusion. If a benzodiazepine is insufficiently effective, the phenothiazine levomepromazine can be used instead or in combination with it. Occasionally, it is necessary to employ phenobarbital or propofol, both being highly sedative as well as antiepileptic. Phenobarbital is given as an initial dose of 100–300 mg, followed by continuous infusion of 600–3,000 mg/24 h, both subcutaneously, but if given by infusion does not mix with most other drugs, necessitating use of a second syringe pump. Propofol has to be given by intravenous infusion and has a very rapid onset of action (about 30 s) and a short (5 min) duration of action, making it theoretically possible to adjust the level of sedation very closely to individual requirements. In practice, it is all but impossible to achieve the ideal of a patient who, having been agitated, is enabled to calm but conscious.

Pain

If pain has not been a problem earlier in the illness, it is unlikely to be so as death approaches. A dying person may not be able to report pain directly, but if they appear restless or uncomfortable and a reversible cause such as a full bladder or rectum has been ruled out, it is appropriate to try an analgesic. The route of medication can continue as before if a gastrostomy is in situ, but without it, most patients will require a change from oral to parenteral. Paracetamol can be given rectally and may be all that is necessary. Morphine is effective in the management of pain, breathlessness, and nocturnal discomfort long before the terminal phase of the illness [27]. If the oral route is no longer possible, it can be given by subcutaneous injections or by a subcutaneous infusion from a portable syringe driver.

If the route of administration is being changed, or one opioid is being changed for another, care should be taken over the dose conversion (see Table 8.1). For instance, a change from oral (or per gastrostomy) morphine to subcutaneous morphine involves a halving of the daily dose, but all such ratios are individually very variable, and doses may subsequently require upward or downward adjustment according to response. A change in the type of opioid is only needed if a stronger agent is needed, such as a change from codeine or tramadol to morphine, or there is evidence that analgesia is not being achieved without adverse effects such as persistent drowsiness or myoclonus. In this case, oxycodone is frequently used as the first alternative to morphine.

Fentanyl and buprenorphine are opioids that are available as transdermal preparations, the latter being more suitable for patients who have not used an opioid previously. These have the advantage that they depend neither on oral intake nor injections but are best for stable pain because of the long delay (up to 23 h) in establishing and in recovering from steady-state blood levels. However, for patients with significant renal failure, there is the additional benefit that the metabolism of these drugs is affected less that of other opioids.

A patient who has gained particular analgesic benefit from a nonsteroidal anti-inflammatory drug (NSAID) can have it continued by suppository (e.g., in the form of naproxen or ketoprofen) or by continuous subcutaneous infusion using a syringe driver. Ketorolac will mix in a syringe with morphine, but if, as is usually the case, other drugs are also required, it is more reliable to give the NSAID rectally.

Conclusion

Care at the end of life is one of the most important activities we can be involved with. It is not only the sole opportunity we ever have to ensure that a person leaves this world without distress but also shapes an experience that resonates powerfully with those left behind who loved the one who died. In their recollection of the person they have lost, their thoughts will over time turn more to the memories of healthier and more active times. Their own attitudes toward serious illness in themselves and in others, and toward healthcare and its practitioners, will be powerfully shaped by the quality of dying they perceive their friend or relative to have been afforded and the extent and the sensitivity of the communication they received during this phase of the illness.

The content of this chapter, therefore, has not just been about the clinical care of an individual but constitutes a public health initiative that has the potential to shape opinion and behavior across generations. It is significant that over half of the complaints received by British hospitals have been found to relate to end of life care and that the great majority of these center on failures of communication [28]. It may feel as if our efforts are concentrated on someone who will soon be past. In fact, they are shaping the fears and hopes of the patients of the future.

References

1. Bromberg MN, Liow M, Forshew DA, Swenson M. A time line for predicting durable medical equipment needs for ALS/MND patients. Proceedings of the 9th international symposium on ALS/MND. Munich: International Alliance of ALS/MND Associations; 1998.
2. O'Brien T, Kelly M, Saunders C. Motor neurone disease: a hospice perspective. BMJ. 1992;304:471–3.
3. Aboussouan LS, Khan SU, Meeker DP, Stehnach K, Mitsumoto H. Effect of non-invasive positive pressure ventilation on survival in ALS. Ann Intern Med. 1997;127:450–3.

4. Henry C, Seymour JE. Advance care planning: a guide for health and social care professionals. Leicester: National End of Life Care Programme; 2008.
5. Fries JF, Everett Koop C, Sokolov J, Beadle CE, Wright D. Beyond health promotion: reducing need and demand for medical care. Health care reforms to improve health while reducing costs. Health Aff (Millwood). 1998;17:70–84.
6. Wilkinson AM. Advance directives and advance care planning: the US experience. In: Thomas K, Lobo B, editors. Advance care planning in end of life care. Oxford: University Press; 2011. p. 189–204.
7. Hinton J. Which patients with terminal cancer are admitted from home care? Palliat Med. 1994;8:197–210.
8. Davison SN, Simpson C. Hope and advance care planning in patients with end stage renal disease: qualitative interview study. BMJ. 2006;333:886–90.
9. Calman KC. Quality of life in cancer patients – an hypothesis. J Med Ethics. 1984;10:124–7.
10. McCoubrie RC, Davies AN. Is there a correlation between spirituality and anxiety and depression in patients with advanced cancer? Support Care Cancer. 2006;14:379–85.
11. Neudert C, Oliver D, Wasner M, Borasio GD. The course of the terminal phase in patients with amyotrophic lateral sclerosis. J Neurol. 2001;248:612–6.
12. Thomas K, Sawkins N. The gold standards framework in care homes training programme: good practice guide. Walsall: Gold Standards Framework Programme; 2008.
13. The Liverpool Care Pathway for the Dying Patient. Liverpool: Marie Curie Palliative Care Institute. http://www.liv.ac.uk/mcpcil/liverpool-care-pathway/. Accessed 8 Sept 2012.
14. Hockley J, Watson J, Oxenham D, Murray SA. The integrated implementation of two end-of-life care tools in nursing care homes in the UK: an in-depth evaluation. Palliat Med. 2010;24:828–38.
15. Turner-Stokes L, Sykes N, Silber E, Khatri A, Sutton L, Young E. From diagnosis to death: exploring the interface between neurology, rehabilitation and palliative care in the management of people with long-term neurological conditions. Clin Med. 2007;7:129–36.
16. Edmonds P, Hart S, Wei G, Vivat B, Burman R, Silber E, Higginson IJ. Palliative care for people severely affected by multiple sclerosis: evaluation of a novel palliative care service. Multiple Sclerosis. 2010;16:627–36.
17. Dalal S, Del Fabbro E, Bruera E. Is there a role for hydration at the end of life? Curr Opin Support Palliat Care. 2009;3:72–8.
18. Dy SM. Enteral and parenteral nutrition in terminally ill cancer patients: a review of the literature. Am J Hosp Palliat Care. 2006;23:369–77.
19. Wee B, Hillier R. Interventions for noisy breathing in patients near to death. Cochrane Database Syst Rev 2008; 1:CD005177. doi: 10.1002/14651858.CD005177.pub2.
20. LeBon B, Fisher S. Case report: maintaining and withdrawing long-term invasive ventilation in a patient with MND/ALS in a home setting. Palliat Med. 2010;25:262–5.
21. Jennings AL, Davies AN, Higgins JPT, Anzures-Cabrera J, Broadley KE. Opioids for the palliation of breathlessness in advanced disease and terminal illness. Cochrane Database Syst Rev 2001; 4: CD002066. doi: 10.1002/14651858.CD002066.
22. Simon ST, Higginson IJ, Booth S, Harding R, Bausewein C. Benzodiazepines for the relief of breathlessness in advanced malignant and non-malignant diseases in adults. Cochrane Database Syst Rev 2010; 1:CD007354. doi: 10.1002/14651858.CD007354.pub2.
23. Ventafridda V, Spoldi E, De Conno F. Control of dyspnoea in advanced cancer patients. Chest. 1990;6:1544–5.
24. Latimer EJ. Ethical decision-making in the care of the dying and its applications to clinical practice. J Pain Symptom Manage. 1991;6:329–36.
25. Cherny N, Radbruch L. European Association for Palliative Care (EAPC) recommended framework for the use of sedation in palliative care. Palliat Med. 2009;23:581–93.
26. Sykes NP, Thorns A. The use of opioids and sedatives at the end of life. Lancet Oncol. 2003;4:312–8.
27. Oliver D. Opioid medication in the palliative care of motor neurone disease. Palliat Med. 1998;12:113–5.
28. Healthcare Commission. Spotlight on complaints. London: Healthcare Commission; 2007.

Chapter 9
Carers

Cynthia Benz and Debra Chand

Abstract More often than not, carers remain the mainstay for individuals with long-term neurological conditions, especially when nearing end of life. Carers anchor those they care for throughout the length of a neurological disease, which may swiftly fatal or protractedly uncertain over a long time. Carers work long hours and are adept at multi-tasking. What they most long for is time to rest and recuperate. They invest their best in caring, combining responsibility with sensitivity to needs of others, and offering hope and support. Without carers, hospitals and care homes would be overwhelmed with patients.

Carers and patients undoubtedly benefit from the input of medical and social care professionals who understand the distinct needs, differences, variabilities, challenges and suffering that may destroy not only physical well-being but also alter the personality of some people with certain neurological diseases. The burden of care is heavy for all involved, voluntary and professional. There are tremendous benefits to care-giving whenever professionals work closely with patients and carers, involving the latter as valuable members of a multi-disciplinary team of colleagues, who pool expertise and prize mutual care.

Keywords Carer support • Communication • Bereavement • Coordinating care • Palliative care

Throughout this chapter, you will find direct quotations in italics from individuals with personal experience of palliative and end-of-life care for long-term neurological conditions. They may be patients, carers, or care professionals. These "authentic voices" have shared their experiences in blogs, articles, and face-to-face discussions. Check the websites of the long-term neurological conditions for more recent contributions.

C. Benz, B.Ed. Hons, M.A., Ph.D. (✉)
Multiple Sclerosis Society, National Council for Palliative Care,
and Dying Matters Coaliation, UK
e-mail: cynthia@benzltd.com

D. Chand, B.Sc., MBA
The PSP Association, 67 Watling Street West, Towcester, Northamptonshire, UK
e-mail: debra.chand@pspassociation.org.uk

D. Oliver (ed.), *End of Life Care in Neurological Disease*,
DOI 10.1007/978-0-85729-682-5_9, © Springer-Verlag London 2013

Starting Out

Definitions

It is important to define who features in this chapter: individuals in need of care, many of whom are near end of life, and their carers, who also deserve attention and support. They exist center of stage but often their voices are not heard. Some find it difficult, impossible, unsure how or too occupied to communicate. At best carers and individuals receive support from family, friends, or neighbors who look out for them, take an active interest in their well-being, care for and love them.

The term patient will be used in relation to people receiving direct care from health and social care professionals. Adults who give or receive support and care will be referred to as carers or individuals. A carer is "someone of any age who provides unpaid support to family or friends who cannot manage without this help. This could be caring for a relative, partner or friend who is ill, frail, disabled or has mental health or substance misuse problems" [1]. The term carer should not be confused with a care worker, or care assistant, who receives payment for looking after someone.

Coordinating Care

This chapter focuses on carers of individuals with a long-term neurological condition who interact with care professionals. Their spheres of influence, lived experience, and professional expertise overlap. What carers most want is information and support [2], which professionals are employed to supply. At the same time, carers build up a store of valuable "inside" information about those they care for, so vital to the successful input of care professionals. Carers and care professionals may also discover how caring for the same individuals fosters mutual support, satisfaction, and a good enough ending.

Whenever neurological conditions progress and lives become further interrupted, the overlap of responsibility for care increases. Because long-term neurological conditions are complex, likely to become burdensome, and open to misunderstanding, it is important to tease out what happens where, when, and how in order to assess what does or does not work well and find better ways to enhance care.

Who Cares and Why?

Some 850,000 carers look after people with long-term neurological conditions in the UK. Most never expect to take on a caring role but choose to stay by and offer support when the need for care becomes obvious. The relationship with the individual needing care, other commitments like family and employment, and the age and health of the prospective carer all play a legitimate part. But for many carers, *"it's simply what you do,"* especially if you are a spouse/partner.

> *"I get frightened sometimes about what the future will bring, how I will cope, but for me there are no options. I love him, he's my mate."* [3]

Inevitably some thrive in a caring role while others struggle to juggle the increasing burdens of caring. "Potential carers" may feel unable or unsuited to caring. Some walk away at diagnosis, fearful of what is ahead. When this happens, the caring may be shouldered by aging parents or younger carers at home, children and teens. It is also important to note that some people live alone, without carers, who "self-care" and have nobody other than care professionals for support.

What Is So Different About Long-Term Neurological Conditions?

Whatever the condition, most long-term neurological conditions are generally not well understood or open to misunderstanding by the public, including health and social care professionals unfamiliar with them. Initially people respond with sympathy and support when someone they know is diagnosed with a potentially long-term neurological condition. Yet many who donate money to neurological charities tell collectors about affected family and friends they rarely see. Pictures of people with visible physical disabilities and in a wheelchair tug at heartstrings but never increase the number of visitors offering direct support. Medical "mysteries," conditions with unknown causes and no cure, are uncomfortable to contemplate, let alone live with, especially if they worsen and cause suffering over extended periods of time.

> *"At first everyone was offering to help but many didn't follow through"* because *"it is hard spending time with someone that has a disability or acts 'oddly.'"* [4]

Visible physical impairments are distressing, confusing, and upsetting enough for most people, but more difficult to cope with are "invisible" symptoms that affect thought processes, social skills, and personality in people who look "normal."

> *"He would come out with some strange things and some real shockers,"* which *"left people thinking he was 'weird.'"* [4]

Yet there are unexpected positive responses as well:

> *"I have found Huntington's Disease has been a great filter, some people stepping back and others forward."* [3]

Caring for People with Long-Term Neurological Conditions

What makes caring for people with neurological conditions any different from caring for people with other conditions? Carers are often both surprised and comforted to find that others who care for people with totally different conditions experience similar challenges and react much the same. Yet it is vital not to underestimate the escalating impact of most neurological conditions that are long-term, progressive, and complex, with the potential of altering behavior. Health and social care professionals occasionally confide that caring for neurological patients is very different from what they are accustomed. When pressed, even experienced professionals in end-of-life care confess how helpless they can often feel when faced with the complexities of neurological conditions that are only resolved when death comes.

Typically individuals and carers live with:

- Uncertainties, beginning before diagnosis and continuing throughout the disease progression
- Variability – this may be hourly, daily, weekly, or more periodic
- Complexities that seem exhaustive, almost defy explanations, and tend to bunch together in a raft
- Losses of many types, most of which are inevitable

Knowing the facts is essential, and care pathways aid the organization of care but, for individuals and carers, it all adds up to a lot to live and cope with. Some stereotypes of certain neurological conditions are obvious, but this is not always the case if people experience a mixture of visible and invisible symptoms. Changes in personality and behavior are wide open to misinterpretation. Options need to be kept open, allowing individuals leeway with the overall aim of preparing for the worst and living life to the best.

The Stresses of Caring

Caring for people with long-term neurological conditions is invariably stressful, and anxiety levels escalate the more progressive the condition becomes. By their nature, most long-term neurological conditions behave unpredictably and usually have intractable symptoms that affect an individual's character and responses.

Helen, Melvyn's daughter, remembers her dad *"with a thousand yard grin,"* who, as MND progressed, found that *"every day became one big challenge."* Not only were *"his frustration and feelings of helplessness… incredibly overwhelming for him"* but also for the family as *"MND seemed to have taken over completely"* [4].

However much caregivers want to care, they may become worn down by trying to cope around the clock. The individuals they care for may have experienced a sudden onset of their condition, been sucked into a slow or fast progressive course, or one characterized by periods of relapse and remission, with any stability being intermittent and unpredictable.

Carers can easily become trapped by the demands of constant caring. Significantly, some carers carry out multiple caring roles, some of which are also long-term commitments: they care for other family members, particularly young children, and may support friends and neighbors, too. Other carers have to go out to work to make ends meet. Little wonder that many become desperate for time to rest – and any leisure would be a bonus. The most important unmet need of carers is time away from the home. [2]

Getting It Together

Securing a Diagnosis

Diagnosing any long-term neurological condition is pivotal for individuals and carers. After living with disconcerting experiences of unfamiliar puzzling symptoms, they need to know what is happening and why.

"*The gradual, degenerative symptoms continue*" with people "*seeing the changes so blatantly*" [5].

Neurological conditions are notoriously difficult to diagnose and individuals often wait a long time.

A neurological diagnosis marks a starting point of a journey into newly named but yet unknown territory – see Chap. 3. Its course and ending are uncertain. Communicated well, the diagnosis has the potential to be a significant act of care, the first of many to come. Individuals and carers need to be offered clear and factual information about the condition, available treatments, and prognosis. After an initial diagnosis of Parkinson's disease, this person was rediagnosed with a rare dementia:

"*Fears for the future are heightened in both of us. They roll round in my head at night.*" [6]

Once a diagnosis is made, continuity of contact and establishing good rapport helps to develop an open working relationship between carers and health and social care professionals. Inevitably, individuals and carers will find from the Internet or via personal contact information that may puzzle, conflict, or upset them.

Becoming a Carer

Carers invest in caring the best they can. Their relationships with individuals needing care, other commitments like family and employment, and their own age and health all play a legitimate part in how much care they can give. This commonly happens when Parkinson's disease creeps up slowly to reveal itself fully in older age, by which time many couples, so used to supporting each other, expect to cope with caring. The emotional involvement of carers is significant as it means negotiating with both positive and negative feelings, which jar and conflict.

What begins as a manageable short-term commitment may escalate and become untenable with increasing disability and worsening symptoms. It is not uncommon for partners of young people with multiple sclerosis to experience this and walk away forever.

"He left me earlier this year because he couldn't deal with my increasing disability – it makes the whole bit about 'in sickness and in health' stick a bit." [7]

Carers usually begin their caring in familiar territory, responding to the care needs of those they have agreed to care for. Carers may soon be faced with unfamiliar situations. Repeated acute episodes and/or relentless progression that typify most long-term neurological conditions inevitably impact on carers and push them to their limits. Clearly they need to know what to expect from specific neurological conditions and what outside support is available.

What Support Do Carers Need?

Carers vary in their reactions to diagnosis and how they cope with caring. The spirit of hope shared by many individuals and carers astounds, buoying up reluctant carers, who care by default. What often surprises is discovering an inner resilience that helps to "empower and promote the strengths and resources of patients within their family and friendship networks and their communities" [8]. Resilience grows out of being invested in someone or something. Energy is released when carers adopt a defensive role against a neurological condition whose affects they strive to minimize.

"I hate MND and the sly little way it has of picking on people and stripping them of everything they have." [4]

Carers' resilience is powerfully supportive and tenacious, for it can carry those cared for through to the end. It may also be costly to carers and leave them stripped of resources.

Many carers take pride in what they do and demonstrate high levels of self-sufficiency. Evidence of this comes from a survey, [2] in which one-third of carers reported not needing further information about neurological symptoms and their possible effect on the person cared for or about the roles and responsibilities of health and social care professionals. Inevitably much depends on how manageable the condition is currently and on the carer's aptitude for and experience of caring. The other two-thirds of carers certainly wanted more information, with a few unsure what they wanted. Two other significant facts also emerged: face-to-face communication was preferred to leaflets and hesitancy over who should initiate sharing information. Carers said they did not always know what questions to ask and expected professionals to offer information whereas the professionals expected carers to ask. The need for information never goes away, and communicating it well is an art. It must be clear and easy to absorb, relevant, and offered in a caring way that neither overwhelms nor frightens. In order to pitch the communication appropriately, it helps to check what lies behind the questions actually asked or listen for clues that carers slip into general conversation.

The need for good communication remains constant from diagnosis to death. Quality communication prioritizes the involvement of patients and carers, who usually function as one unit despite assuming different roles. One way to encourage this is getting to know patients and carers during the assessment and planning of care and in this way ensuring that patients, carers, and professionals work together. [2]

Carers' assessments record what carers are coping with and what help they believe will improve things. Assessments aim to establish supportive contacts, like a key worker, often the GP, and liaison with other services so that carers know who to turn to for specific information, especially when needs change. They also help to maintain supportive relationships with professionals. Regular reviewing of records serves to safeguard carers' health and well-being. For example, it notes potential care overloads and which carers look after others in addition to the individual with a neurological condition. It may also warn of future difficulties facing carers of people whose increasing changes in mood and behavior will probably demand extra attention.

Planning starts by establishing current needs and concerns, exploring how to meet them, and reviewing the recent past and its trends in order to prepare for future possibilities. One area of planning covers practical matters such as providing equipment and training in handling it, improving skills in caring, or contributing to decisions regarding treatment. Another key area is contingency planning for care in emergencies. Significant numbers of carers surveyed were concerned that anyone with high dependency needs should receive appropriate care without delay if anything happened to their carers. Setting up out-of-hours helplines or equipment breakdown services was well supported. [2]

Beginning to Share Care

Carers and health and social care professionals jointly focus on providing care that benefits patients as well as possible. At best they complement each other in what they contribute. On a daily basis carers build up a store of valuable "insider" information and experience about the individuals they are caring for, which is vital to the successful input of healthcare professionals.

> *"PSP is such a specialist thing, people don't 'get' it a lot of the time and, do you know what, sometimes you just get so fed up explaining it all, don't you!?"* [5]

Carers gain confidence and strength from being heard when they share their experiences of caring: health and social care professionals gain very honest insights. Respect and mutuality between carers and professionals enhance support and care. Over time care professionals will assume increasing responsibility for both carers and patients whose neurological conditions progress. They will become aware of the contrast between the supportive environment they work in, with manageable caseloads, set working hours, and the benefit of good colleague backup, and the isolation and long hours most carers work with little outside support. Some carers give up work or education to care, with financial implications. Others provide care for more than one person. [2]

The relationship between carer and the person cared for needs safeguarding. Services that make a positive difference allow carers to choose how much they can care and support them to the end. Such services must be comprehensive, for example, meeting the needs of young children also cared for at home, and sensitive to cultural differences, as well as providing breaks for carers, which the majority long for. Nearly two-thirds of carers surveyed wanted more help to get away and recharge. Often they were simply unaware of the services that were available or refused them in case they upset the individuals cared for. [2]

Gale's sister "*didn't accept outside care or support*" even from two specialist charities, one for the condition and the other providing palliative care, and "*went downhill rapidly*" [4].

Interestingly, although overall carers said "the most important unmet need is time away from home," one-quarter of carers reported never needing to take a break. [2]

Coming to Terms with Neurological Conditions

The challenges of supporting patients with long-term neurological conditions are shared by both carers and care professionals. The latter monitor the impact of the condition on patients and carers, including the difficulty of balancing the burdens and rewards of caring-giving, and find ways to "interpret" to patients and carers the contradictions around caring in positive ways. Carers' lived experience of caring in different and complementary ways adds a pragmatic and dynamic dimension. "Their perspective is critical to the care of the patient" [9].

However, not all health and social care professionals who interact with patients and carers have had the benefit of specialist neurology training. Together with carers, they too have to face the reality of a wide and unfamiliar spectrum of neurological symptoms, which has the "capacity to evoke the most negative and despondent attitudes" [10]. At one end lie visible symptoms which clearly display what is malfunctioning and may respond to treatments and palliation. At the other end are invisible symptoms, hidden from sight yet powerful in impact. [2]

Cognitive symptoms that appear to "distort" the personality of patients and affect their behavior are prime examples. They are common in conditions like Huntington's disease and may also develop during the progressive stages of other conditions. Hidden symptoms disquiet because they are unpredictable, rarely controllable, and seem to rob patients of their identity.

"*But now, he's a different man, a different Dad and a different husband.*" [5]

When changes become extreme, communication incoherent or behavior violent, people feel threatened or alienated and, consciously or unconsciously, "step back." This natural "gut level" response to being unable to control the unknown may compromise the quality of care offered. It is easy to unwittingly convey messages that caring is becoming burdensome. What wins through is "good enough" care, backed up with support that keeps a realistic balance, a willingness to learn from experience, and adequate time off. "Good enough" care is kind, has a listening ear, with finely tuned "intelligence" to assess a situation, aided by gentle questions or intuitive response.

Changes of Pace

A Working Relationship

It is striking how adept carers and individuals are at establishing a "working relationship" with their specific neurological condition in which small unwelcome changes become part of daily routines.

> *"It seems this disease is one long series of small losses, tiny changes from day to day that you don't always notice, but then when you look back at what life was like a year ago or five years ago, suddenly the change and the loss can seem huge."* [6]

Any change of pace is unsettling, even a really positive one like going from MS relapse into remission carries uncertainty about how long improvement will last. However, most changes in neurological conditions are synonymous with progression and occur in different ways at any time between diagnosis and death, varying in intensity, speed, and impact.

Rapid progression or relentless decline creates a fluid situation. Carers may never have imagined how such suffering could be endured let alone witness it ever happening to someone they care for and love. Spontaneous recollections of the raw impact of progression may echo on, unresolved for those who cared.

A teenage son remembers *"the first day of a vicious attack my mother had"* and *"the shock of what was happening. The confusion and guilt instantly sank in and left me feeling, at times, almost isolated and afraid of the future – her recovery wasn't certain"* [11].

When lives become disjointed by disease, care needs increase. With patients increasingly at risk, carers face greater vulnerability in caring. What was previously manageable becomes too complex to cope with alone and challenges professionals to "engage fully with carers as co-experts in care delivery" [12].

> *"She needs round the clock attention now, and I am determined that is what she will get, but at what cost to me?"* [6]

Clearly the top priorities are to stabilize patients and support carers.

Caring for people with neurological conditions is never straightforward, and carers' stress levels rise the more progressive or complex the condition becomes. In addition to physical symptoms like pain, incontinence, and mobility, there are often problems with communication as well as disease-specific losses, many of them multiple. The unpredictable element that typifies neurological conditions is unnerving. Although carers know "*it is the disease that is changing him/her...*" [3], the reality of constantly living alongside it can cause distress and grind carers down. This is particularly true when faced with cognitive dysfunction, passivity, depression, behavioral problems with aggression, or certain dementias that leave patients to "slowly deteriorate to a point where there can be little or no meaningful exchange" [13].

Coping with neurological disease is also demanding psychologically with questions like "why me?", emotionally with feelings of sadness over losses, fears for the future or anger from frustration, and socially because of isolation and not fitting in. There is also a spiritual dimension to do with meaning and transcendence, and what exists to anchor and support at such times. Throughout it all uncertainties abound about what to expect next and how to manage.

Progression

The impact of a change of pace is obvious from watching what happens to the patient. It may be a close call in the case of sudden and rapid progression, an emergency admission to hospital or hospice, or an intervention to manage the cumulative effects of slow progression, especially if aggravated by a common infection. Negative and unwelcome, the effects on the health and well-being of patients deserve total care – body, soul, and spirit. Health and social care professionals need training, skills, and practice in caring for patients with chronic conditions who develop acute medical needs and to be up to speed with medical ethics to guide best practice. Unfortunately not all professionals have adequate experience of long-term neurological conditions, which is a serious concern. [14]

Progressive episodes often leave patients and carers reeling from "irrecoverably shattering experiences" [15], the consequences of which may reverberate. For instance, the patient care load may be doubled, and the carer may be left with inadequate support. It is wise not to underestimate how shaken carers often are after witnessing the powerful effects of progression. The worst-case scenario is a sort of downhill slide as carers struggle to come to terms with the fact that although they have given of their best, nothing can avert the course of the disease. Experiencing the reality of progression evokes emotional responses that threaten to overwhelm in ways that neurological facts rarely do. At the same time carers usually become physically exhausted from relentless increases in burdens of caring, which can leave patient and carer feeling isolated. Yet, resilience, combined with strong bonds of relationship, may enable carers to carry on beyond their normal capabilities.

Although caring for carers is good practice, it may not always occur in reality as carers are not top priority, the care they need is seldom a medical emergency, and they may not recognize they need support at the time as:

• An understandable and inevitable consequence of struggling on single-handedly
• Some may have asked for support and not received it, and perhaps their request has not even been heard

- Others refused support because they felt they were managing
- Others would welcome support but were held back by patients who did not see the necessity of having outside intervention
- Support for carers needs funding

Giving appropriate support takes time and demands a mixture of approaches from people who are well-trained, insightful, and most importantly caring and trustworthy.

Reviewing the Situation

Whenever neurological conditions progress and lives become further disjointed and interrupted, there needs to be a greater overlap of caring between patients, their carers, and health and social care professionals. "Best practice" care is about being proactive and supportive. To do this successfully calls for the expertise and resources of a full complement of professionals from different disciplines of health and social care, and palliative care especially, in order to work together as a multidisciplinary team – see Chap. 6.

Once the patient is stabilized, reassessment is needed, not limited to matters of health but including a complete overview of the situation. Sometimes medical treatment to relieve distressing symptoms, for example, is easier to achieve than other areas of concern that affect quality of life for patient and carer. Assessment is not merely a fact-finding exercise, particularly in the aftermath of progression: more an opportunity for an act of caring, with the promise of more to come. Simply being there, able to listen and absorb calmly, takes the sting out of distressing experiences, and is one way to demonstrate support. Patients and carers need time to mull over the implications of current experiences of "their" neurological condition. Total care in action assumes responsibility for many kinds of patient and carer needs.

Experienced health and social care professionals know the sort of pathways that lie ahead and the benefits of considering possible options in order to be better prepared. Conversations that touch on how people feel, their hopes and fears, suffering and meaning, and spiritual support take on new significance toward end of life. Everyone reacts differently to experiences of loss, how to recognize and face them, and find a way through. People often assume that talking about the future will be difficult and uncomfortable and are surprised when conversations seem to happen almost spontaneously and leave them feeling relieved.

Acknowledging the Burdens of Care

Caring for a member of the family, friend, or neighbor is a voluntary arrangement, normally made by choice and possibly already in place before diagnosis, so caring for someone with a long-term condition becomes a serious commitment. In practice, "long term" varies according to the condition. The average life expectancy for people with neurological conditions ranges from under 2 years with MND through to near normal for many with Parkinson's disease or relapsing and remitting MS, who may never know that their condition could affect their lifespan. Average life expectancy is a rough and ready guide, fraught with exceptions and constant uncertainty. So long-term caring can prove burdensome, especially if it lasts decades, involves cognitive and behavioral changes, and the carers are aging themselves.

Facts about carer burden speak for themselves. However much caregivers want to care, they may become worn down by trying to cope around the clock. In one study, 95 % of carers experienced constant strain, 92 % lost sleep because of worry, and 84 % reported feeling unhappy and depressed [2]. "Compassion and support fatigue" builds up, leaving many carers too exhausted to carry responsibilities for care and likely to opt out [13]. Carers generally experience lower than normal levels of quality of life and physical health, with even poorer levels of mental health linked with distress and depression. These can exceed the threshold for mental health disorders in situations where those cared for have dementia and behavioral problems and refuse to cooperate with carers [2, 15]. Little wonder that relationships are eroded.

> *"There may be a warm breathing body, but the personality of the one with terminal disease seems absent: I lost him/her years ago."* [9]

Practicalities, Support, and Advance Planning

It sounds straightforward to "put one's house in order," but it takes time, involves careful organization, and some heart-searching.

> *"When I was diagnosed, I said to my wife, 'whatever happens we'll find a way of coping'. I still believe we can, from a practical point of view, but I never realised that it would be so difficult psychologically."* [6]

It is standard good practice to encourage everyone – patient and carer – to make a will, keep finances in order, and have personal papers and documents readily available so that someone else can take over easily. Achieving this brings peace of mind.

Many carers take a pragmatic approach to planning care. They know what services and support they need to care well and what happens when they are unable to access them. Those who are confident about managing care at home would still welcome greater backup support and investment in contingency planning. In particular, carers want to avoid hospital admissions, welcome hotline help, and getting support at short notice for highly dependent people. [2]

Carers rarely have any choice over what caring role they take on or type of care they have to provide, whatever their circumstances at home. Securing support for children and other dependent family members eases the load. As care becomes more demanding, the most important unmet need of time away from home becomes more difficult to arrange. There may be opposition from the person being cared for, the carer's own reluctance over letting others take over, or dependency issues. Carers from different cultural and faith backgrounds often have specific concerns. [2]

Carers experience great relief when they do share the challenges and load of caring. Contact with other carers on Internet forums, by telephone, or face to face in carers' groups can be amazingly supportive. The weight of constant practical caring can be lifted by negotiating alternative care, such as professional care at home, or where the individual is moved into a care home, hospice, or hospital as appropriate. If the transition is left too late, carers will be overexhausted to negotiate it smoothly. Whenever people are cared for temporarily or permanently in other settings, carers' roles change. Caring becomes more about overseeing and taking responsibility for their loved ones to get good care.

Letting go of "hands-on" caring will seem like a loss to some carers and a great relief to others. It allows carers opportunities to recover their strength and renew relationships with family and friends that will be supportive. The best outcome is when carers have more time and relaxation. The presence and touch of a carer no longer troubled by burdens, stress, and strain may be a balm to the patient and provide anchorage. Personal relationships may deepen and be enriched by closeness, a shared history, and strong emotional attachments, the reality of which is familiar and comforting. Equally, patients may be angry about being "sidelined," adding a level of guilt for stressed carers, which may be eased by the tactful intervention of professionals.

Advance care planning differs from general planning because it anticipates the possibility that a person's health may deteriorate in future (see Chap. 9). Often it is patients themselves, perhaps together with carers, who send out clues suggesting it is something they want to talk about – "At the end of my life…" or "I've been thinking that I'd like to be cared for in…" Carers are often party to such discussions. It really depends on the patients. It is a very positive step to take and share with those most closely affected.

Loss

Experiencing loss has the potential to erode or enrich. Carers have firsthand experience of how neurological conditions create losses, some more bearable than others. Coping with loss of health depends on what care is on offer, background, personality and experience, previous circumstances, outlook, and spirituality. Each individual is likely to have a hierarchy of losses most feared. Loss of health may trigger a series of other losses that commonly affect self-confidence, relationships, work, and social life.

Carers face their own losses, too, especially when they are no longer seen as spouse, partner, or lover but simply as carers. Losses may be expressed with sadness, a normal and healthy reaction, or its flipside emotion, anger. How losses are grieved over varies from person to person, on the circumstances surrounding the loss, and cultural expectations. Losses can affect health negatively and are associated with poor appetite, disturbed sleep, despondency, and depression, all of which are well-recognized problems that many carers struggle with. Yet there are "opportunities for growth, healing and support for both patient and family . . . even while they are coping with countless difficulties and sorrows as the patient's disease progresses" [9].

One such opportunity is "bereavement needs assessment," which aims to minimize the risks associated with loss and prioritize support for people who are vulnerable. [16] Some people respond to loss in strongly emotional ways that overwhelm, feel their distress will never go away and that life will never be the same again. Others face loss with emotions firmly under control and get on with life in clearly considered pragmatic ways. Coping well requires a resilient approach that balances emotional, social, and practical responses to loss. Unlike denial, resilience is about facing the real impact of loss, expressing appropriate emotional reactions in safe ways, attending to practicalities, and seeking consolation from caring and supportive relationships. As people differ in what inner resources they have to cope, it is vital that care professionals do not leave vulnerable carers to manage alone. Exploring with carers what support will help – practical, social, psychological, and/ or spiritual – provides benefits all round. Support and affirmation enable people to acquire coping skills and develop resilience to stand them in good stead for the future.

Anticipatory Grief

This is not an uncommon fleeting thought in everyday life and may happen spontaneously to anyone. Patients, carers, family, and friends may experience anticipatory grief, alone or together, and sometimes long before death comes, like a rehearsal. It is often triggered by awareness of deterioration or progression in the patient's condition. At such times, people tend to talk more openly about what is happening and reflect on journeys of many losses, past, present, and future, including their own. Letting anticipatory grieving just "be" and moving on when ready seems most appropriate. It is one way of taking stock and being prepared for the inevitability of death for everyone. It neither hastens nor delays death. If some people become unduly upset, professional support like bereavement counseling should help.

Involving Carers as Partners in the Multidisciplinary Team

Carers have been described as "the lynchpin of community care" [17] because of their vital role in giving individuals the care they need. They deserve respect and an opportunity to become partners in care with health and social care professionals. Partnerships of coworking can only exist within a relationship of trust where all appreciate the value of pooling expertise that is different but complementary. For each "expert patient," there can be an "expert carer" with a wealth of "local knowledge" of the patient. By comparison, training and experience give professional carers "cosmopolitan knowledge" [18].

However, carers have no automatic right to be involved in a multidisciplinary care team. The care team has a primary duty to accommodate patients' preferences for end of life, which may affect what carers can contribute. Carers choose to care for various reasons, which are not open to scrutiny, so professionals tend to opt for the safety and manageability of a known team. Even with security checks in place, some fear that including carers will hinder efficient professional practice. In fact, carers often have very high expectations of professional care and carefully monitor how professionals use their knowledge and skills as proof of their trustworthiness. Because "carers lose trust in professionals more rapidly than relatives do" [19], some are reluctant to entrust the care of loved ones to others. The development of trust between professionals and carers is not automatic. Only professionals who notice carers, want to get to know them, and are responsive to their needs and wishes earn their allegiance as co-colleagues.

Dying, Death, and Bereavement

Would it surprise you if… were to die in the next few months? [20]

This is a common question among professionals when a patient appears to be approaching a terminal phase. [21] How easy is it to provide an answer for people with long-term neurological conditions? The chronic and acute experiences, unpredictabilities, and variabilities of neurological conditions have already deeply influenced the lives of patients and those close to them. Accommodating illness rather than health has affected all aspects of everyday living, "activities, roles and relationships and the very meaning of life itself" [9]. When death is on the horizon, even after months, years, or decades of chronic illness, patients, carers, families, and friends focus on life in new ways. Everyone struggles to come to terms with the present and how to face challenges around dying.

Neurological disease with its potential to develop complex symptoms that disable and cause physical, psychological, cognitive, and behavioral suffering and deterioration, often with intractable pain, is possibly more variable than most. Some deaths associated with long-term neurological conditions are sudden and unanticipated. There would also seem to be some characteristic patterns of dying – rapidly terminal for some people, old or young, or a prolonged wobbly decline. Others simply slow down in old age, their deaths possibly hastened by frailty and disabilities. For each individual "death won't be hurried. It has its own rhythm" [22]. What matters now is how to prepare to say good-byes, affirm what is positive and supportive in life, and secure good care. "In the face of death there is no second chance" [12].

Quality Care at End of Life

It is possible to illustrate very simply what contributes to good end-of-life care by considering the input from patients, carers, and healthcare professionals. The aspects of care at this time include the following.

Patient's Awareness of the Future

Becoming prepared combines practical planning and coming to terms with the inevitability of death. Although "these are unchartered waters for single-craft only" [22], patients will usually turn to close carers to accompany them as far as possible. Getting on with practicalities may begin early for people who characteristically face life's realities full on or who are advised on diagnosis of a neurological condition like MND that time is likely to be short. It can also be a frustrating time:

> "I'm unable to do what I want any longer and I don't like others making decisions for me!" [6]

Yet individuals frequently express concern about leaving the people they love and care about and how they will manage. It helps when carers and individuals share the writing of a will, deciding preferred priorities for care or advance decisions to refuse specific medical treatment at end of life. Carers are often the natural first choice as attorneys who will take decisions on behalf of patients should they subsequently lose capacity. Carers sometimes find themselves challenged by individuals who wish to become organ donors. Once the practicalities are settled, individuals and carers can focus on more personal preparations, together or singly. The closeness and compatibility of relationships may strengthen during that bittersweet time before death. Or the reverse may happen – a moving apart in anticipation of separation. It is certainly an emotional time, the full impact of which carers may feel later.

Experiences of Care

What anchors people and gives them courage at end of life are all the experiences of care they have invested in, feel nurtured by, and return to for succor. Carers and individuals often serve as anchors to each other. Carers may personify anchorage. There is a timelessness about anchors, which is perhaps why good care always counts even if the preferred carer cannot be there to make it perfect. Good relationships, past or present, top the list and may include pets as well as people. Other anchors include significant places like gardens and countryside, music and literature, customs and culture, a recognition of things that touch the soul, like spirituality, or a chosen faith that gives support in life, death, and beyond.

Communication and Support from the Caring Team

Whatever the setting in which end-of-life care is offered – at home, in a hospital, hospice, or care home – it is a unique opportunity to put into practice "total care" with honest communication. This will include the carers as much as the patient. At end of life, carers usually become more involved as patients weaken and possibly lose capacity. It is about easing the transition from life to death with sensitivity, understanding, and respect for the dignity of individuals at their end and also being mindful of those left behind who need support, too.

Increasing Care Burdens Toward End of Life

Carers will certainly have wondered, only fleetingly perhaps, how and when the end may come. Their lived experience of neurological conditions remains as unpredictable at the end as it did at diagnosis. Caring for individual fluctuations, variations, and uncertainties that seem "never ending" and not knowing what's in store may make everyday living surreal. As "professional care alone cannot expand to meet the needs of all the dying and bereaved" [8], they are "in for the long haul," unless, as in the case of motor neurone disease, death is likely to come soon. Compared with cancer, caring for people with any long-term neurological condition "is by no means less eventful or stressful and . . . their problems may be even more severe or wearing since the duration of care is frequently longer and unpredictable, interspersed with frequent periods of great uncertainty" [15].

The impact on carers of living alongside people whose long-term neurological condition then becomes terminal adds a new dimension. Death is surrounded with overwhelming issues and concerns, spiritual and practical, about what lies ahead for those who die and those left behind. Frequently many years of repeated exacerbations and remissions have already taken their toll on carers, who now face caring for loved ones with an unpredictable and possibly prolonged decline toward death. Carers may struggle when watching rapid deterioration and suffering that leaves them feeling helpless. Coping with lack of rest, anxieties, and endless demands and preparing for future eventualities calls for "delicate care networks" to be in place. [15]

Carer Buffers

Near the end of life of a patient, a carer's role undergoes significant changes. The autonomous role of carers frequently safeguards the private and personal relationships with those they care for. In many instances, carers have not only kept their families intact but also involved them in the home care team. Carers need buffers, and the most resilient carers turn to extended family and friendship networks for support. Smaller families, especially if socially independent or isolated, may be more at risk. It depends on what carers can cope with and what support is available and successfully accessed.

Reassessing Carers' Roles at End of Life

Caring for patients with complex care needs near death is demanding and often intensive and usually requires additional involvement from the care team. Relinquishing personal care and management to professional carers may be a relief but carers often feel that a close bond has been severed. Yet professional caregivers should not underestimate how much carers still have to offer that is uniquely valuable, to patients and to the team. For example, carers often recognize and interpret subtle changes in reduced energy, engagement, and mood in those they care for as imminently terminal much earlier than do nurses or doctors.

How carers and patients react to the approach of death also changes the dynamics of relationships. Some families close ranks and keep everything very private, while others gather family and friends around them and contact distant relatives. One positive practical outcome occurs when individuals who previously expected carers to care single-handedly finally let them access support networks or agree to accept professional or specialist palliative care. They may also wish to have final contact with those especially close, caring and cared for, including children and young people who may need help to face death and grieve positively. Some carers are still young themselves. Seeing someone so well-loved deteriorate and die in difficult circumstances is a weighty burden to carry at any age. It brings comfort and strength to share that last journey supported by a wider community of people, known, trusted, and loved. Sadly the opposite may also happen, when family and friends argue and fight, unable to resolve differences, and never become reconciled.

Preparing Carers for the End of Life Journey

What lies ahead challenges everyone, not least carers, whose experience may already be so "fraught and fragmented" that "they feel inadequate for the task of being carers" [23]. When a dying person nears end of life, careful preparation and support provide much needed anchorage for everyone involved. What helps most is warm and open contact with a care team that communicates and connects well. Its members initiate conversations with carers and patients associated with issues around care and dying. Integral to total care is responsiveness to needs and being ready to accompany both patient and carer from start to finish, "and then some." It is important that carers know that professionals are obliged to offer life-sustaining care and how that might work in practice.

Carers need guidance on how to cope well in changing circumstances and reassurance that they may still contribute as part of the care team. They may learn new skills and approaches in cooperation with professional carers who pay regular visits. Even if their input is not as "hands on" as before, carers need to hear how uniquely valuable their presence and support are. "The presence of capable and willing carers makes possible a range of options and choices such as being cared for and dying at home" [12]. Overall care burdens may increase but remain manageable because good practical support exists and the end is in sight.

Communication

Sometimes patients and carers feel as if they are being kept in the dark about what is happening toward end of life. This may be their first experience of dying. Communication made with respect and kindness compensates when words fail. Nonverbal communication may be more honest than words. Communication skills are especially important when sharing emotionally sensitive information with carers or responding to their questions about what to expect, when, and why care may be given or withdrawn.

> *"Conversations about her deterioration only occurred when I instigated them. They were not forthcoming – I had to instigate them. I wanted to know what stage she was at. Sometimes I noticed changes but the nurses kept saying that she wasn't dying. I got really angry because I knew she was in that process."* [24]

When care professionals take the initiative to communicate, it spells genuine care and respect. Professionals who are able to relate to patients, carers, family, and friends as equals and communicate care as fellow human beings, not simply professionals in role, are remembered with gratitude long afterward.

Information About Dying

The most vital information carers must know is when those they have been caring for are approaching end of life. Despite striving daily to cope with physical deterioration, increasing disability and frailty, patients and carers may well miss obvious changes that are related to deterioration. Even familiar patterns of repeated admissions to hospital may not warn them that emergency intervention cannot continue indefinitely. Sometimes carers and patients with long-term neurological conditions have never been told to expect death.

For example, people diagnosed with Parkinson's disease or multiple sclerosis are usually advised that their lifespan will most probably be close to normal, unless they experience progressive disease, and even then, in some cases, death is not on their radar. Yet the consequences of not knowing are grim as one husband testifies.

"H died after an extended and horrible period of illness. The death is recorded as due to bronchopneumonia and multiple sclerosis. In a few months, she suffered from practically every symptom recorded as attributable to multiple sclerosis. She was terrified about what would happen until mercifully she apparently stopped being able to comprehend the future. In her last weeks she perhaps even stopped registering pain. At no time were H and I made aware that progression of MS could be as severe or as rapid as it turned out to be. Nor that the condition was likely or perhaps certain to be terminal. Perhaps I should have been able to infer that but I didn't." [25]

There are obvious sensitivities to take into account as the patient has a right to receive information rather than the carer. However, from early in the disease progression it helps to clarify with patients whether information can be shared openly with carers. Most patients choose to include their carers or other significant people in such discussions. However, nobody has a right to participate without the patient's agreement or by prior legal arrangement, such as taking on Lasting Power of Attorney for Health and Welfare if the patient does not have capacity.

End-of-life discussions focus on the sort of care patients want to receive and their specific wishes about interventions such as "do not attempt cardiopulmonary resuscitation," or artificial feeding or hydration. They need to understand that whatever is done will maximize benefit and minimize harm. If such discussions distress the patient, the doctor is not obliged to share information the patient does not want to hear. In that case the doctor will ask if the patient would like someone else, like the carer, to be informed and, with the patient's permission, will share the information. However, if the patient does choose to have the conversation, with or without the carer present, the doctors are obliged to share the facts honestly according to their professional opinion. [26]

The Right Place to Die and the Most Appropriate Care

Where people want to die is important, not only to them but also to carers, family, and friends. Dying is a personal "taking leave of life" that deserves privacy and intimacy, where busyness does not interfere. Most people say they want to die at home yet over half die in hospital. This poses a dilemma for carers, who are rarely asked what they prefer. Many carers fear they will not cope with a home death and are anxious about getting the right medical care and backup. Some also wonder how they will manage to live in the same place after their loved one has died. Careful discussion about the issues involved – practicalities around caring as well as the emotional issues of coping with the death itself – may be facilitated. In this way, planning can develop with the flexibility to change according to circumstances.

Carers' Reactions to What They Witness at End of Life

Carers would dearly like to help those they love when they experience distressing symptoms like intractable pain or breathlessness. In fact, the vicarious suffering of carers may precipitate patient admissions to hospital or hospice.

Pain, in particular, is a widely accepted metaphor for illness: carers regularly over-estimate pain as more intense and severe than patients do and consequently become upset and stressed. Since 50 % of people with multiple sclerosis and motor neuron disease experience pain, adequate and lasting pain control is a key issue. Carers feel especially helpless seeing someone in pain, and many wish they could share the suffering and carry the load. Other long-term problems like incontinence, loss of appetite, behavior, and dementia often coexist and become more severe and difficult to manage as death approaches and consequently the weight of caring increases.

This invariably impacts negatively on carers physically and psychologically. They may not manage to cope any longer or become so immersed in trying to care that they totally override their own needs, sometimes ignoring serious health concerns. It matters that "their problems and losses are not discounted simply because they have not raised them as issues. All problems experienced by carers, either in isolation or in combination, should be sensitively sought out, acknowledged, and, where at all possible, addressed" [15]. Reaching out and taking the initiative seem to be a recurrent issue between health and social care professionals, patients, and carers. When carers so closely involved with loved ones at death's door fail to recognize their own needs, they certainly deserve care.

Involving Carers in End-of-Life Care: A Personal Challenge for Carers

"No one actually spoke to us about death and dying. And we never actually asked anyone." [25]

Carers and patients who do not realize for themselves that end of life is near need to be told. Supporting a loved one at end of life is personally challenging. Even when carers have been closely involved in advance care planning and know what patients wish to happen at end of life, no one knows how it will actually happen. Many people have never witnessed an actual death and fear it.

Those who have seen death may also struggle, especially with their own demise. *"What is distressing is that she knows what is happening to her. She used to manage a care home and she is frightened"* [6].

Carers are often unprepared for the rapidity and severity of death and may discover that *"the process of dying was more difficult than the prospect of death itself"* [27].

Without good care and support in place, patients and carers do become overwhelmed and distressed. *"Parkinson's is robbing my Father of his body and mind… having to watch him every other day getting worse and worse is killing me slowly."* And 2 days later, *"he is dying… how do I stay strong?"* [6]

Balancing Roles and Relationships

Care professionals are familiar with the tension that often exists between the roles people take on and who they actually are. This tension can act as a challenge to respond within role and with a human touch. A similar tension also exists for carers, even if they do not recognize it, especially at end of life. Carers offer the best care they can and give much of themselves. What they most desire is that their loved ones should retain their dignity and have a "good death." Care professionals have a responsibility to prepare both patients and carers to face death honestly despite their vulnerability by offering them emotional support, practical information, and open communication.

Emotions

Dying is an emotional experience: emotions well up unbidden and catch people unawares. The deaths of a spouse or child are viewed as personal tragedies. Feelings are natural human responses to different kinds of experience. People feel sadness when they anticipate or experience loss and often shed tears, anger when frustrated and helpless, and fear when facing the unknown. Some carers also feel depressed, guilty, or lonely while others experience hope and peace to the end. Support from understanding people who are not phased by emotions is really helpful.

Channels of Communication and Support

One very practical and successful way of improving communication in a hospital setting is via a carer's diary left at the patient's bedside. It might include the carer's comments on clinical practice and observations on care given, expressions of thanks and appreciation as well as personal reflections on dying, death and facing bereavement. Diaries allow carers to engage more meaningfully in end of life care and their availability to clinical staff allows concerns to be addressed immediately. [28]

Dying and Death: "How Long Now?"

Carers, and patients too, are often specifically concerned about recognizing signs of approaching death. They want to know how long dying takes, when and how to let go, and who should be present at the death. They usually look to the care team for reassurance and insights such as *"Knowing when it's going to happen is not significant – it's more about knowing when you've had enough"* [26].

Last Words

At the end of life, when the connection with one significant person nears its end, communication is cherished and remembered. Patients, carers, families, and friends may wish to express their deepest thoughts and struggle for words. Yet deep and meaningful communication can be more than words: listening, looking, watching and waiting, smiles and tears, smells, touch and taste, openness, silence, and presence also communicate. Carers want to be with their loved one to the last, together with family and closest friends. Often great significance is placed on last words. At death many people call for a chaplain to "say some words" or simply to be present with them at the bedside.

A Good Death

Dying may be universal but each death is uniquely individual. Possibly the greatest pain a carer can feel is to be alone and unable to help, only able to watch and wait until suffering ends in death.

> *"I find myself wishing she was gone, that her pain and distress will end . . . this disease is very, very cruel."* [4]

A good care team understands the concept and practice of total care and knows what palliative care intervention is appropriate at every stage. Subtle shifts in mood and decline are recognized, reassessed, and acted on. Supporting patients and carers by addressing their concerns and needs, physical, psychological, emotional, social, and spiritual, enables them to find meaning each step of the way. Facing the reality of what is happening even in the bittersweet time of death's approach may have a touch of deep richness and joy when families stay together, take time to reminisce, reflect and say goodbyes, and help to achieve "a more peaceful death."

Bereavement and Grieving

Bereavement has been described as the loss of someone or something precious, which can never be recaptured. Death draws a timeline in the experience of those who grieve – before and after. There are so many variables to come to terms with: unexpected or anticipated death, death in old age after a long and satisfying life, death of a child or young person, accidental death, or because of ill-health. Sudden and unanticipated deaths are the most difficult for those bereaved to accept. How people die really matters – the more peaceful, the better.

Bereavement is when people initially register their loss and feel bereft. Deaths of people with long-term neurological conditions have deep roots, leaving carers and family with great needs and ambivalent feelings, such as release and relief or devastation and guilt. Sadness and grief are often accompanied by depression, distraction, sleeplessness, restlessness, anger, or guilt. Grieving is a painful process of accommodating the reality of the loss and adjusting to a different world with one new empty space.

"I believe that grieving is nothing to be ashamed of. It is part of the healing process and it cannot be avoided, no more than the healing process can be speeded up." [6]

It is easy to say that support helps but much more difficult to contribute even one small comfort that might make a difference to any mourner. Presence and listening skills are equally valuable and potentially empowering before and after death. The ability to stay with people without trying to resolve their struggles makes a positive difference in helping them find new coping skills.

One wonderful example is a caring MNDA visitor *"who has time for you day and night. She's very much part of the family and you can talk to her about anything. She helped my son cope after losing his granddad and, without her support, I know my son and I would be in a far worse state"* [4].

There is a strong and beneficial link between the support carers received before the death that "has a profound influence on bereavement following the death of the patient" [9]. Carers who have gone through the process of anticipatory grief also seem to have benefit compared with those who have not. It is also important to attend to the general health of carers. Recovering from physical exhaustion, stress, and anxiety takes time and carers may not be able to grieve fully until they feel fitter.

Contact with a tried and tested care professional often works successfully but may be difficult to maintain long enough after the death. Sometimes carers find bereavement counseling helpful because they have specifically chosen to seek support and have more control over how long they want the contact to last. Talking through experiences of caring, losses and death takes time. Sharing painful facts and feelings needs the safety of understanding, acceptance and no criticism. Long periods of caring, prioritizing the needs of others, and experiencing personal loss leave carers barren and needing nurture before they gradually readjust and discover a fresh purpose in living.

Conclusion

The lived realities behind this chapter will always remain ongoing and unresolvable. They challenge all who encounter carers of individuals with long-term neurological conditions to help them care the best they can. Carers are not only anchors for those they care for, they are also an inestimable resource within the community despite their lack of formal training and professional status.

The primary responsibility of health and social care professionals is to patients, but carers come a close second for their unique role accords them both autonomy and vulnerability.

Their fortitude and resilience, often caring single-handedly, is admirable. It is also important to "be aware of the potentially fragile emotional state of carers" [2] because many are prone to wear themselves down because of stress, anxiety, and overwork.

The "hardware" of care is clearly prescribed yet often woefully underfunded in terms of cash, services, pathways, and personnel. It is important to put in place all the practical supports, guidance, good practice, comprehensive services, and trained care personnel of every speciality. "How we care for the dying is an indicator of how we care for all sick and vulnerable people. It is a measure of society as a whole, and it is a litmus test for health and social services [29]."

Yet it is the "software" that makes all the difference in the world to patients, carers, and to care professionals themselves. Carers and health and social care professionals share the potential to be invaluable "software." Not having answers and not being able to change the unchangeable never stops them from trying to give of their best. They rejoice at being able to give "significant acts of care" and prize small victories. Their hallmarks are to be real, honest, open, and supportive. It shows in the ways they care by establishing good rapport, communicate, listen, and can be trusted.

There is also a need for champions at the coal face who care proactively and support in ways that are gentle and tough by turn. Such champions keep their finger on the pulse and stay the course.

Best practice care takes responsibility for addressing all kinds of patient and carer needs and understands that mutual support, expressed through appreciation and affirmation, has worth that lasts to the end.

References

1. Carers Trust. www.carers.org.
2. Research Initiative for Long Term Neurological Conditions. www.ltnc.org.uk.; Jackson D, Turner-Stokes L, Harris J, et al. Support for LTNC carers, particularly those with multiple caring roles: an investigation of support needs and the cost of provision. London: Department of Health; 2011.; Jackson D, Williams D, Turner-Stokes L, et al. How do carers of people with long term neurological conditions experience the provision of replacement care? London: Department of Health; 2011.
3. Huntington's Disease Association. www.hda.org.uk.
4. MND Association. www.mndassosciation.org.
5. PSP Association. www.pspeur.com.
6. Parkinson's UK. www.parkinsons.org.uk.
7. Comment from private correspondence from a young person with multiple sclerosis to Cynthia Benz, author.
8. Monroe B, Oliviere D. Resilience in palliative care – achievement in adversity. Oxford: Oxford University Press; 2007. p. 2–7.
9. Panke JT, Ferrell BR. The family perspective. In: Hanks G, Cherny NI, Christakis NA, et al., editors. Oxford textbook of palliative medicine. 4th ed. Oxford: Oxford University Press; 2010. p. 1437–44.
10. O'Brien T. Neurodegenerative disease. In: Addington-Hall JM, Higginson IJ, editors. Palliative care for non-cancer patients. Oxford: Oxford University Press; 2001. p. 44–55.
11. MS Trust – mystory. www.mstrust.org.uk.
12. Payne S. Resilient carers and caregivers. In: Monroe B, Oliviere D, editors. Resilience in palliative care – achievement in adversity. Oxford: Oxford University Press; 2007. p. 93.

13. Maddocks I, Brew B, Waddy H, et al. Palliative neurology. Cambridge: Cambridge University Press; 2006. p. 37–41.
14. Report by the Comptroller and Auditor General. HC (House of Commons) 1586 Session 2010–2012. Services for People with Neurological Conditions - Full Report. London: The Stationary Office; 16 December 2011. Section 3:3.16 on page 38 and 3.20 on page 40. National Audit Office. www.nao.org.uk.
15. Koffman J, Shaw P. Informal carers of dependents with advanced disease. In: Addington-Hall JM, Higginson IJ, editors. Palliative care for non-cancer patients. Oxford: Oxford University Press; 2001. p. 2–238.
16. Relf M, Machin L, Archer N. Guidance for bereavement needs assessment in palliative care. 2nd edn. London: Help the Hospices; 2010. www.helpthehospices.org.uk.
17. Nolan M, Ryan T. Family carers, palliative care and the end of life. In: Gott M, Ingleton C, editors. Living with aging and dying – palliative and end of life care for older people. Oxford: Oxford University Press; 2011. p. 170–80.
18. Harvath TA. Establishing partnerships with family caregivers: local and cosmopolitan knowledge. J Gerontol Nurs. 1994;20(2):29–35.
19. Schoot T, Proot I, ter Meulen R, de Witte L. Recognition of client value as a basis for tailored care: the view of Dutch patients and family caregivers. Scand J Caring Sci. 2005;19:169–76.
20. Thomas K, Sawkins N. The gold standards framework in care homes training programme: good practice guide. Walsall: Gold Standards Framework Programme; 2008.
21. Turner, J. Article: "Death won't be hurried. It has its own rhythm." In the Opinion section on page 23 of The Times. 17 March 2012.
22. Benz C. Patients' perspectives. In: Addington-Hall JM, Higginson IJ, editors. Palliative care for non-cancer patients. Oxford: Oxford University Press; 2001. p. 198–209.
23. Arber A, Hutson N. Carers of people with primary malignant tumour: are their information needs being met? Br J Neurosci Nurs. 2010;6(7):329–334. (Oct 2010) www.bjnn.co.uk.
24. Black J. National Council for Palliative Care. Difficult conversations – making it easier to talk to people with dementia about the end of life. London: National Council for Palliative Care; 2011. p. 18. www.ncpc.org.uk.
25. Helped by Dr. Coles' Article - Letter from H's husband. New Pathways Magazine. Issue 51, 2008. p. 11. www.msrc.co.uk.
26. Randall F, Downie RS. Palliative care ethics – a companion for all specialities. 2nd ed. Oxford University Press: Oxford; 1999.
27. Michael. Talking Point - We Weren't Prepared for the End. New Pathways Magazine. Issue 54, 2009. p. 48. www.msrc.co.uk.
28. Mel McEvoy, Nurse consultant in cancer and palliative care. North East Strategic Health Authority. The Clinical Network September 2011. www.theclinicalnetwork.org.
29. Department of Health. End of life care strategy: Executive Summary, point 6, page 2. London, 15 July, 2008. Only available as a download from www.dh.gov.uk/publications.

Chapter 10
Future Developments in Care: National Strategy and Commissioning

Claire Henry and Beverley Hopcutt

Abstract An integrated approach to commissioning is essential for the development of services, and this needs to be steered by national strategy for long-term conditions and end of life care. A commissioning model can draw together a number of key components that enable an integrated service to be delivered for the individual, their family, and carers and ensure that care is delivered in a dignified and respectful way by the right person, in the right place, at the right time.

This chapter focuses on policy in England, and although some aspects are unique to England and Wales, the principles of commissioning good quality end of life care would apply equally to any other developed country. Often the key to delivery is having the correct infrastructure in place which is built on good communications between all parties with the individual and their families/carers at the center. This all needs to be supported by a trained and competent workforce which needs to be included as part of the overall commissioning.

Keywords Commissioning quality end of life care • Long-term neurological conditions • Workforce • Measuring the quality of EOLC

> **Case Study: Northamptonshire's Palliative Neurology Service**
> Northamptonshire's specialist palliative care service has been offering a palliative neurology service for patients with rapidly progressing neurological conditions such as MND and MSA and has developed over the past 15 years. It consists of a multidisciplinary team of palliative medicine consultants, physios, and OTs as well as having links with a range of allied services that

C. Henry, RGN, PgDip, B.Sc. (✉)
National End of Life Care Programme,
3rd floor, St John's House, East Street, Leicester, Leicestershire, LE1 6NB UK
e-mail: claire.henry@eolc.nhs.uk

B. Hopcutt
Therapy Service, Central Manchester University Hospitals NHS Foundation Trust, Manchester, UK

D. Oliver (ed.), *End of Life Care in Neurological Disease*,
DOI 10.1007/978-0-85729-682-5_10, © Springer-Verlag London 2013

can be called upon when needed. The team holds clinics at the two hospices based in the north and south of the county as well as making frequent visits to people in their own homes or nursing homes.

The service supports about 50 patients with neurological conditions such as MND from diagnosis and MSA, PSP, prions disease, and CBD from the time they reach a more palliative stage through to end of life care. The initial assessment aims to be holistic and is followed up on a regular basis.

The service came into being because patients with MND were receiving no specialist support and conventional statutory services were simply too slow. Dr. Fiona Wiseman, Consultant in Palliative Medicine states, "They just couldn't respond quickly enough to people's changing needs. For instance, they would be waiting weeks and weeks for equipment by which point it was often too late."

The current service places the emphasis on being proactive and therefore avoiding the crises that so often lead to hospital admissions and unnecessary cost and distress. "We try to get things in place before they become a problem," says Fiona. "And what we have been able to demonstrate is that this has enabled people to stay in their preferred place of care and to die where they want to die."

As a result, it is rare for anyone in the county with a progressive neurological condition to be hospitalized. The service has also proved popular with patients and carers. A recent survey indicated people felt reassured by the support and expertise that is on hand and reported they were getting things like specialist equipment in a timely manner. Carers also appreciated the support they received.

Fiona Wiseman states: "They are living with conditions that are fluctuating and changing rapidly and they really appreciate that there is a specialist team on hand who will have seen this before and can say, 'here's a different approach that might help.'" She feels that the team's presence also enables patients to begin the process of advance care planning at an earlier stage. "ACP is rarely done at one sitting but whenever the occasion arises," explains Fiona. "But because we've developed a rapport we can gently explore what information they want and when is the best time to talk this through."

National Strategy

Commissioning of quality end of life care for long-term neurological conditions (LTNCs) has been supported by a number of different national strategies:

The Long Term Conditions National Service Framework (LTC NSF) [1] was published in March 2005 after more than 2 years of preparation. It was produced with a high level of engagement with people with LTNCs, their carers, and the voluntary sector in addition to the typical involvement of a reference group of experts.

As a new style of NSF, it did not set national standards with national targets for implementation but instead defined 11 quality requirements (QRs) with evidence-based markers of good practice for local implementation within a 10-year delivery period.

The Long Term Conditions Model [2] described a tiered approach to the delivery of health and social care support to people with chronic conditions. This had been published shortly before the NSF and reinforced some of the key principles in the NSF, including:

- Patient empowerment through information to self-manage their condition
- Making informed choices about their care
- The need for an adequately equipped generic workforce to meet the nonspecialist needs of people with LTCs with access to a more specialist workforce
- Services for those with more complex needs

It also emphasized the importance of avoiding admission to hospital through improved management of the LTC, as did the NSF.

This model applied equally to the management of end of life care (EoLC) in LTNCs as it did to earlier stages of the condition. This highlighted the need for the specialist workforce – in this case, palliative care – to work collaboratively with the neurological and rehabilitation workforce and to skill up the generalist primary health care and social care workforce delivering day-to-day care and support.

Quality Requirements of the NSF: Within the LTC NSF, Quality Requirement nine addressed palliative care, stating that

> People with long-term neurological conditions nearing the end of their life are to have access to a range of palliative care services as and when they need them, to control symptoms and offer pain relief, and to meet any personal needs they may have [1].

This statement was made in 2003 and predates the National End of Life Care Strategy but did coincide with the document "Building on the Best" [3]. The aim had been to improve quality of care at the end of life for cancer and noncancer patients and enable more patients to live and die in the place of their choice, but most specialist palliative care services were dedicated to people with cancer. The only LTNC likely to be accepted by hospices and other specialist palliative care services was motor neuron disease, mainly because it was a rare rapidly progressing condition and so unlikely to make significant demands on resources.

The key to implementing QR9 was rolling out the use of three end of life tools that had been developed for cancer patients but that are applicable to other conditions. The tools are:

- Preferred Priorities of Care, which is an example of an advance statement as a patient-held document. It is used to facilitate and record patient choice in relation to end of life issues [4]
- The Gold Standard Framework, which was initially developed for use in primary care settings so that people approaching the end of life can be identified, their care needs be assessed and a plan of care with relevant agencies put into place [5]

- The Liverpool Care Pathway, which is an evidence-based framework to support those delivering care to the dying patient and their relatives in the last days and hours of life, in a variety of settings [6]

The evidence-based markers of good practice for QR9 focused on the delivery of improved end of life care through the collaboration of specialist and generalized services and workforce development via on the job and more formal education. These are the following:

- Marker 1: Specialized neurology, rehabilitation, and palliative care multidisciplinary teams and providers work together to provide care for people with advanced LTNCs.
- Marker 2: People with advanced LTNCs have access to specialized and generalized palliative care services which support them in their home or in specialized setting according to their choice and needs and in line with national best practice guidelines and specialized neurological and community rehabilitation services provide support, advice, and training for all staff delivering palliative care in the community.
- Marker 3: Staff providing care and support in the later stages of a LTNC have appropriate training. This should ensure that neurologists and neurorehabilitation teams are trained in palliative care skills. It should also mean that all staff providing care for people in the advanced stages of neurological illness are trained in both the management of LTNCs and palliative care.

A policy research program, funded by the Department of Health, accompanied the NSF and aimed to expand the evidence base and support implementation. The LTNC NSF research initiative [7] was launched in late 2005. A total of ten studies were commissioned with one focusing specifically on end of life care. This study found that in these conditions the problems and needs are similar in nature and severity to those experienced by people with cancer and that better management of these symptoms is likely to improve their quality of life and reduce the carer burden [8].

The End of Life Care Strategy [9], published in July 2008, aimed to improve access to high-quality care for adults approaching the end of life. This care was to be available wherever the person is, whether that is home, care home, hospital, hospice, or somewhere else.

The strategy addressed a number of key areas, including:

- Raising the profile of end of life care and changing the attitudes to death and dying
- Strategic commissioning to provide an integrated approach to planning
- Care planning to assess the needs and wishes of the individual and agree a care plan
- Coordination of care
- Rapid access to care and support 24/7
- Delivery of high-quality services in all locations

- Using an integrated care pathway in the last days of life
- Involving and supporting carers
- Education and training and continuing professional development
- Measurement and research to monitor the care given and develop further services

Later reports emphasized the involvement of palliative care in LTC:

- Long-term conditions and end of life care remained high on the agenda as part of the *NHS Next Steps Review* [10] led by Lord Darzi where end of life care was a core component and every regional health authority had work streams addressing these agreed priorities. In some cases this included neurological conditions. The NHS Operating Framework which lays out the important priorities for the NHS 2009–11 [11] continued to incentivize good quality EoLC, reinforcing the use of recognized tools such as PPC.
- *High Quality Care for All* (2008) [12] reinforced the content of the NSF. It emphasized the importance of EoLC for all, regardless of underlying condition, and the need for collaborative teamwork to ensure that individuals' specific needs were met. To this end a series of good practice documents have been produced to highlight condition-specific issues and management. The EoLC in advanced neurological disease good practice guidance was published in 2010 [13].

Commissioning policy has also changed markedly over this period. When the NSF was launched, primary care trusts were charged with its implementation with an exhortation to engage with social services in order to achieve the desired improvements in longer-term care and support. Individual controls of certain aspects of the social care budget for personal care through direct payments were at the pilot stage.

However, the current landscape is very different as there is now even greater emphasis on personalization of social care budgets with people with a LTC holding their own real or virtual individual budget which enables them to commission their social care. It has been suggested this could be extended to aspects of health care funding.

At an organizational level, PCTs are being phased out and the vision of *Liberating the NHS* [14] is giving GPs greater local control as clinical commissioning groups with local authorities identified as key decision makers. An NHS Commissioning Board will oversee the process and have responsibility for commissioning more specialist national/regional services. This policy is still evolving, and its impact is unclear, but there remains an ongoing commitment to supporting people with LTCs and providing high-quality EoLC.

Commissioning a Person-Centered Service

An integrated commissioning model (Fig. 10.1) has been suggested [15]. Each element of this approach, which centers on the individual and their carer, focuses on the six steps of the end of life care pathway. The importance of the workforce

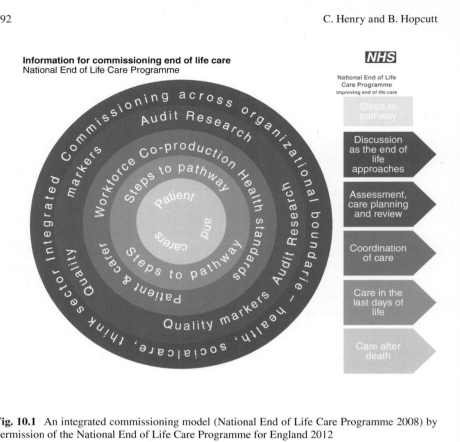

Information for commissioning end of life care
National End of Life Care Programme

Fig. 10.1 An integrated commissioning model (National End of Life Care Programme 2008) by permission of the National End of Life Care Programme for England 2012

and the need to measure quality is then highlighted, and it suggests integration between health social care and the third sector across all geographical boundaries.

From a commissioning perspective, it is vital that local strategies are underpinned by robust financial and operational plans that set out how these aims will be achieved and the investment and timescales required. As end of life care services will, of necessity, span a range of needs (not solely health-related) and involve a range of potential service providers, strategic planning and service coordination needs to be undertaken jointly with partner local authorities, informed by sound joint strategic needs assessment (JSNA) processes.

An integrated commissioning model (National End of Life Care Programme 2008)

Effective commissioning for end of life care should include the following key characteristics:

- Be based on need
- Forecast demand
- Be based on partnership

- Promote and assure equality of access
- Build from pathway-based specifications
- Embed choice

Funding

Long-term conditions tariff development has included work on costing a year of care, an approach which is better suited to long-term conditions which require ongoing and often multiagency care rather than one-off episodes, predominantly relating to health care. The MND Association has developed and trialed a year of care pathway for an individual with advanced disease, and this approach is transferable to other LTNCs [16].

Lead commissioners for LTNCs may wish to consider developing local applications of this approach to support people with advanced neurological disease. It can also be used to inform the development of local pathways for individual budgets and personal health budgets as part of the personalization agenda.

Funding also needs to support a joined-up approach to the commissioning and delivery of care. It is acknowledged that the statutory provisions for joint or pooled health and social care budgets are underutilized. Person-centered care needs to transcend the organizational boundaries that can so often build in delays to the commissioning and delivery of timely care – no more so than when the individual enters the advanced stage of a LTNC. There are examples that demonstrate it is possible, by collaborating around the individual, for health and social care to overcome these barriers and streamline and integrate processes.

Case Study: North Manchester's Individual Budget Funding Pilot
In north Manchester a new innovative funding mechanism has been developed for people with motor neuron disease using individual budgets. The scheme aims to make funding available to the patient when it is needed and avoid bureaucratic delays as their condition deteriorates.

The pilot was introduced a year ago after someone with MND who was using his individual budget to employ two friends as carers encountered problems because of the delays between being reassessed and receiving a new, increased funding package.

"Each time the patient's needs changed a care manager had to revisit and carry out a new assessment and then present this to the commissioning panel for approval, by which time his condition had often changed again," explains Cath Roberts, Clinical Lead, Community Occupational Therapy, with University Hospital of South Manchester. "Basically the process was too slow for somebody whose rapidly progressing condition caused them to become almost fully dependent on carers in the space of 3 months."

Under the new system, the first assessment of someone diagnosed with MND gives the green light for the full funding package to be allocated – although it will only be released on a graduated basis, depending on the individual's needs.

Each time there is a significant change in the person's condition, the health professional on the ground fills in the necessary paperwork and forwards it to the care manager who can then release the funding when it is actually needed.

So far the new system has been used twice and has involved patients whose care package is managed by the care manager on their behalf, using care agencies. In each case the process has worked smoothly with extra funding being made available promptly to fund a new, more intensive care package when the person's condition has changed.

Transitions occur throughout the long-term conditions journey, and this is true of the end of life care elements of the pathway. These can be between providers across sectors and both formally and informally. It is vital that end of life care is commissioned using an integrated pathway approach that incorporates transitions such as from children and young adults to adult services. As the individual's condition deteriorates, the focus of care may start to shift from purely focusing on cure to including elements of palliative treatment. Over time, the ratio will start to alter as the focus shifts increasingly to palliative and end of life care – see Fig. 10.2 [17].

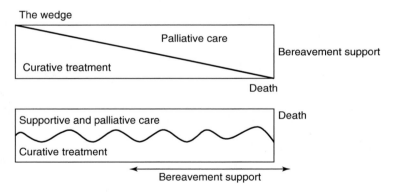

Fig. 10.2 Palliative care over time (Taken from Ref [17])

End of Life Care Pathway: The Individual's Perspective

The end of life care pathway is key to commissioning good person-centered care. And communication is fundamental to good commissioning of end of life care. At both the strategic and individual level, the pathway of care can only really start when the individual, their carers, and professionals start to communicate.

Stage 1: Discussion as the End of Life Care Approaches

It is vital that health and social care professionals know how to initiate conversations. It is imperative that these professionals have the correct training which should be ongoing. Training should include experiential learning as communication skills need to be practiced on a regular basis to ensure that the professional is confident and competent to have these conversations.

At this stage, it is important that professionals have guidance to help them identify when a person is starting the transition into end of life care. One useful question to ask is: "Would you be surprised if Mr X was to die in the next year/6 months?" If the answer is no, that would be an indication that the professional should start to consider end of life care needs. Other tools include the prognostic indicators which have been developed by the Gold Standards Framework team.

Stage 2: Assessment and Care Planning

This is a key aspect of both EoLC and LTNC management. People with LTNCs value an integrated approach to assessment, and this is a key recommendation of QR1 of the NSF. This is particularly important when an individual has advanced disease and does not have the energy to repeatedly tell their story and outline their needs to the plethora of health and social care professionals involved in their case. The emotional burden of advance care planning cannot be underestimated, so it is vital that this is coordinated by a key professional supporting the individual to make their ACP (the care coordinator as expounded in QR1). This role, valued by people with LTNCs in QR1, is also vital for quality EoLC.

This is underlined by the findings of one of the baseline NSF research studies which showed that the individual was more likely to experience integrated care if there was a care coordinator [18]. It is important that this role is recognized as part of the service specification. This helps to ensure that information about assessment and the care plan is shared across all agencies and the right care (in terms of the individual's expressed choices about EoLC) is delivered in the right place at the right time.

To support the individual to devise an effective care plan that can meet complex needs and contain effective contingency plans requires a workforce with the right level of communications skills and knowledge of the ACP process. Care plans may include an advance statement, advance decision to refuse treatment, or a lasting power of attorney.

Case Study: Woman with Parkinson's and Dementia
Mrs. Pearson* was an 81-year-old widow with advanced Parkinson's disease and dementia.

She had been admitted to the local district general hospital from her own home because she was no longer swallowing safely and had lost weight. Initially the hospital team was going to arrange for a PEG feeding tube to be fitted. Debi, one of the hospices clinical nurse specialists in palliative neurology, was asked to see Mrs. P by the general medical consultant responsible for her care.

Debi met the lady with her two daughters. She learned that Mrs. Pearson had been failing mentally over the last few months and latterly had been barely coping because of her dementia. She had been an active member of her community and was involved in charity work all her life. It was clear on assessment of capacity that she had no insight into her problems and could not express any opinion about a PEG feeding tube.

Debi contacted Mrs. Pearson's GP, and his impression of the patient over the past few years was invaluable to understanding the wider context.

The consultant arranged a team meeting with Mrs. Pearson's two daughters to decide what to do next. Meanwhile Debi had done a literature search and found that PEG feeding in dementia did not usually confer any benefit and should be considered only in exceptional circumstances. In reaching a best interests decision, the daughters also indicated that their mother would not have wished to be dependent on anyone for her care and would have fought against any form of life prolongation at this stage.

The decision was taken not to fit a PEG feeding tube and to care actively for her other needs. If any problems arose from aspiration, these would be treated on a symptomatic basis.

Over the next few days, Mrs. Pearson developed silent aspiration, and she became drowsier but not breathless and did not show any signs of suffering. It was agreed to transfer her to St Catherine's Hospice for terminal care. She died 5 days after admission. She was very comfortable throughout and showed no signs of distress.

Debi's intervention meant that Mrs. Pearson's capacity for the decision was properly assessed. She also obtained the daughters' views on what they believed their mother would have wanted and acted as a liaison between hospital and community by speaking directly to the GP.

As a result, Mrs. Pearson was spared the possibility of life-prolonging treatment which it seemed she would not have wanted. Debi was also able to provide objective evidence that PEG feeding in dementia rarely confers any benefit. Finally, Mrs. Pearson was enabled to die peacefully with the wishes of her daughters clearly heard and respected.

*Patients' personal details have been changed to preserve the patient and family's anonymity

Case suggested by Dr Colin Campbell, Consultant in Palliative Medicine, Saint Catherine's Hospice, Scarborough

Another key skill is the ability to support the individual to navigate their way around the health and social care system and access the services of their choice/need as set out in their care plan. Those commissioning services will need to ensure there is time for care coordinators to deliver this integrated care across organizational boundaries and to overcome practical issues such as incompatible IT systems and lack of shared documentation.

It is also important that the needs of carers are acknowledged. The NSF research program demonstrates that the burden of caring for an individual with advanced neurological disease should not be underestimated. Yet two research studies showed that only 52 % [19] and 43 % [20] of those caring for someone with a LTNC had been offered a carer's assessment. Building the offer of a carer's assessment into the contract will help to make this routine practice.

Stage 3: Multidisciplinary Care

High-quality EoLC which meets the many complex needs of those with advanced neurological conditions is dependent on effective multidisciplinary and multiagency working. There is the potential for a number of specialist practitioners to be involved (for instance, neurologists, palliative care, and neurorehabilitation) as well as generalist practitioners who have a wealth of expertise about caring for that individual (for instance, the GP, DN, formal carers, and social worker). It is important that this care is properly coordinated. Someone needs to be able to recognize when specialist input is required and who to approach for that input. Networks of clinicians are helpful as in some cases the solution to the management of certain symptoms may involve collaboration between specialists such as palliative care and neurorehab. Contracts need to allow sufficient time to develop and use these networks.

Stage 4: Care Delivery in Different Settings

People with LTNCs live in a wide range of settings. Some may have moved into supported living facilities and residential and nursing homes to better meet their care and support needs. It is important that high-quality EoLC is available in all care settings, and indeed there are many examples where support staff have been trained in EoLC workforce competences. Commissioners can influence workforce development through their contracts with these different providers.

Stage 5: Last Days of Life

The point comes when an individual enters the dying phase. It is vital that staff can recognize that this person is dying, so they can deliver the care that is needed. How someone dies remains a lasting memory for the individual's relatives, friends, and the care staff involved. This can be expected but in some cases will be sudden. For commissioning, it is important that all organizations have an end of life care pathway in use such as the Liverpool Care Pathway.

Case Study: Woman with MS

Lynne was a 48-year-old single woman with advanced multiple sclerosis, living in a nursing home. She had deteriorated overall in the last few months and was now bedbound with contractures of her legs and had a suprapubic catheter. Her speech was barely audible, and she was susceptible to choking. She went on to have two hospital admissions because of aspiration pneumonia.

Lynne discussed her options with Sandie, a clinical nurse specialist in palliative neurology at her local hospice, and chose to come in to the hospice and have a PEG feeding tube fitted. Over the next few months, Sandie supported Lynne in the nursing home, and Lynne was again able to enjoy her favorite brass band music through her headphones. Indeed, with Sandie's help, she even managed to get to a brass band concert and meet individual band members after the performance.

Once again, however, she began to have aspiration chest infections. One day, Sandie broached the subject of how much Lynne understood about her poor prognosis and what she would like to see happen from this point. Discussion was slow because of Lynne's speech problems, but over two or three visits, she was able to say clearly that she did not wish to be admitted to hospital again. Indeed, she did not now wish her life to be prolonged at all. It was agreed that Sandie should speak to her GP and to the nursing home staff to ensure that if she got a further chest infection, she would be managed at home.

Two weeks later, she became "chesty" once more. A syringe driver was started with Buscopan to dry up chesty secretions. Lynne was very comfortable using this, and gradually over the next week, she became weaker, and it was evident that she was now dying. On what proved to be the last day of her life, Sandie visited Lynne again and found her to be a little agitated as her breathing had become more rapid. After discussing the matter over the phone with one of the hospice consultants, Sandie added medication to the syringe driver to slow the breathing and to relieve any distress Lynne might be experiencing. This proved very effective, and Lynne died peacefully with nursing home staff with her.

What this case study clearly shows is the importance of involving patients and families in discussions about where and how the patient is to die. As in all palliative care, empowering the person to make informed choices for themselves is infinitely preferable to someone else doing things to them without their views being heard.

In spite of her increasing speech difficulties, Lynne was helped to talk cou-
rageously about her deteriorating health and to recognize that she would die
in the near future. Sandie sensitively sought out from Lynne what was important to her and what sort of person she was. She supported her to make choices
which fitted with her own wishes. Lynne's views and wishes were central to
the care provided by Sandie.

*Patients' personal details have been changed to preserve the patient and
family's anonymity

Case suggested by Dr Colin Campbell, Consultant in Palliative Medicine,
Saint Catherine's Hospice, Scarborough

Stage 6: Care After Death

Good end of life care does not stop at the point of death. When someone dies, all
staff need to follow good practice, which includes being responsive to family wishes.
The support and care provided to relatives will help them cope with their loss.
Commissioning needs to ensure that support for the bereaved is an integrated part of
the care pathway. This can include support from volunteers through to professional
counseling. But the key is an assessment undertaken by a professional to ensure the
individual gets the correct support. This may be especially important if the death
was unexpected.

Workforce

It is important that commissioners give proper consideration to the workforce as
part of the overall commissioning process. If the workforce is not confident and
competent, the services that have been commissioned will not be delivered. The
strategy divides the end of life care workforce into three basic groups:

Group A – Specialist end of life care workforce
Group B – Frequently deal with end of life care
Group C – Occasionally deal with end of life care

All members of the multidisciplinary workforce supporting people to live with
LTNCs need to have the knowledge and skills to enable them to support the individual and their family on the EoLC pathway. This is not something that can be left
to specialists in palliative care. All practitioners need the knowledge and skills outlined in the *Common core competences for health and social care workers working
with adults at the end of life* [21]. Effective delivery of care in line with the EoLC
pathway is dependent on the quality of the workforce. Commissioners may wish to

use these competences when contracting with services such as neurorehabilitation, reablement, generic care, and nursing providers to ensure that the workforce is competent to deliver all aspects of EoLC. It is also important to build strong foundations during the earlier stages of the disease, before the onset of communication and/or cognitive difficulties, when people with LTNCs will find it easier and have the capacity to make informed decisions and express those choices as an equal partner in ACP.

All areas and organizations involved in end of life care will need to consider staff training needs across the whole of the end of life care pathway, particularly in relation to the four key areas:

- Assessment
- Advance care planning
- Communication skills
- Symptom management [9]

All staff working in general and specialist services should have the opportunity to develop their knowledge and skills, including an understanding of neurological conditions and the collaborative approach and joint working that are essential to achieve this.

A range of workforce initiatives have been developed to support end of life care delivery, including e-learning modules. Some of these modules focus on advanced neurological conditions. For more information, please visit www.endoflifecareforadults. nhs.uk/workforce.

Education opportunities might include:

- Attendance at study days
- Other formal teaching
- Interdisciplinary education between teams, which can be another effective way of sharing knowledge and learning
- "Informal" initiatives, which can be a very valuable learning experience with information being cascaded through teams

Good face-to-face communication between health and social care professionals and patients and carers is fundamental to the provision of high-quality care.

Measuring Quality for Now and the Future

Measuring quality should be integral to all commissioning. The specifications need to have clearly identified outcomes which are measurable. These may be national, such as quality markers, or local measures such as commissioning for quality and innovation (CQuINS). These could include the usage of Liverpool Care Pathway, response time to calls when an individual needs help in the community to the number of people dying in the place of their choice.

There are several national measures that have been developed that can be used to measure quality. These include national quality markers, which were developed in collaboration with the Strategic Health Authorities end of life care leads and the Department of Health. These follow the steps of the end of life care pathway and are also divided by settings. The top ten quality markers are:

1. Have an action plan for the delivery of high-quality end of life care that encompasses patients with all diagnoses and is reviewed for impact and progress
2. Institute effective mechanisms to identify those who are approaching the end of life
3. Ensure that people approaching the end of life are offered a care plan
4. Ensure that individuals' preferences and choices, when they wish to express them, are documented and communicated to appropriate professionals
5. Ensure that the needs of carers are appropriately assessed and recorded through a carer's assessment
6. Have mechanisms in place to ensure that care for individuals is coordinated across organizational boundaries 24/7
7. Have essential services available and accessible 24/7 to all those approaching the end of life who need them
8. Be aware of end of life care training opportunities and enable relevant workers to access or attend appropriate programs dependent on their needs [21]
9. Adopt a standardized approach (the Liverpool Care Pathway or equivalent) to care for people in the last days of life
10. Monitor the quality and outputs of end of life care and submit relevant information for local and national audits

The quality and productivity key performance indicators and the NHS operating framework measure of the proportion of deaths in usual place of residence that includes home and care homes are valuable to commissioners. The NICE Quality Standard for End of Life Care for commissioners and service providers builds on both these national measures.

It is also important to consider ways of capturing the individual's experience of how services are delivered. Helpful tools that can be used are real-time feedback; there are several companies providing this type of tool, as well as questionnaires such as VOICES, which is completed by the bereaved relative.

Nationally available datasets are an important source of information for commissioning. A LTNC dataset has been developed which includes a subset of data for EoLC. Although not nationally mandated, it is available for use as a reference dataset on the Information Centre website [22]. Collection of this dataset, which consists of seven core items plus another 20 additional items, could be built into the service spec supporting the local contract for LTNCs.

The National End of Life Care Intelligence Network in England provides useful datasets, including local profiles, which enable commissioners to compare themselves to other areas with similar demographic profiles.

Commissioning for Now and the Future

As has been shown, commissioning end of life care for individuals with LTNCs and their families and carers is complex. It is vital this is centered on the individual and their family with built-in quality measures and opportunities for individuals and their families to provide feedback. It also needs to be supported by a trained and competent health and social care workforce. It is critical now and for the future that commissioning works to achieve an integrated service. As Dame Cicely Saunders says, "How people die remains in the memory of those who live on."

References

1. Long term conditions national service framework. London: Department of Health; 2005. Available from: http://www.dh.gov.uk/en/Publicationsandstatistics/Publications/Publications PolicyAndGuidance/DH_4105361. Accessed 28 Oct 2011.
2. Department of Health. Supporting people with long term conditions. An NHS and social care model to support local innovation and integration. London: Department of Health; 2005.
3. Building on the best. London: Department of Health; 2003.
4. Lancashire & South Cumbria Cancer Network; National Preferred Priority for Care Review Team. Preferred Priorities for Care – National End of Life Care Programme Version 2.2. 2007. Available from: http://www.endoflifecareforadults.nhs.uk/tools/core-tools/preferredpriorities-forcare. Accessed 28 Oct 2011.
5. Thomas K. Caring for the dying at home. Companions on the journey. Oxford: Radcliffe Medical Press; 2003.
6. Ellershaw J, Wilkinson S, editors. Care for the dying: a pathway to excellence. Oxford: Oxford University Press; 2003.
7. Research Initiative for Long Term Neurological Conditions website. [Internet] Available from: http://www.ltnc.org.uk/. Accessed 27 Oct 2011.
8. Leigh N, et al. Defining the palliative care needs of people with late-stage Parkinsons disease, multiple system atrophy and progressive supranuclear palsy. Research Initiative for Long Term Neurological Conditions website. [Internet] 2011. Available from: http://www.ltnc.org.uk/. Accessed 27 Oct 2011.
9. National end of life care strategy for England. London: Department of Health; 2008. Available from:www.dh.gov.uk/en/Publicationsandstatistics/Publications/PublicationsPolicyAndGuidance/DH_086277. Accessed 27 Oct 2011.
10. Darzi L. High quality care for all: NHS next stage review final report. London: Department of Health; 2008.
11. The operating framework for the NHS in England 2009/10, 2010/11. London: Department of Health; 2008, 2009.
12. High quality care for all. London: Department of Health; 2008.
13. Improving EoLC in neurological disease: a framework for implementation. Leicester: National End of Life Care Programme; 2010. Available from: http://www.endoflifecareforadults.nhs.uk/assets/downloads/FC_2010_17____neurology_report___Final_draft___20110208.pdf. Accessed 27 Oct 2011.
14. Liberating the NHS: legislative framework and next steps. London: Department of Health; 2010.

15. Information for commissioning end of life care. Leicester: National End of Life Care Programme; 2008. Available from: http://www.endoflifecareforadults.nhs.uk/publications/commissioningeolc. Accessed 27 Oct 2011.
16. MND Year of Care Pathway. MND Association website. [Internet] 2009. Available from: http://www.mndassociation.org/for_professionals/sharing_good_practice/mnd_year_of_care.html. Accessed 27 Oct 2011.
17. Payne S, Seymour J, Ingleton C. Introduction. In: Payne S, Seymour J, Ingleton C, editors. Palliative care nursing: principles and evidence for practice. 2nd ed. Maidenhead: McGraw-Hill Press; 2008. p. 6.
18. Bernard S, Aspinal F, Gridley K, Parker G. Integrated services for people with long-term neurological conditions: evaluation of the impact of the national service framework. Research Initiative for Long Term Neurological Conditions website. [Internet] 2010. Available from: http://www.ltnc.org.uk/. Accessed 27 Oct 2011.
19. Jackson D, et al. How do carers of people with long term neurological conditions experience the provision of replacement care? Research Initiative for Long Term Neurological Conditions website. [Internet] 2011. Available from: http://www.ltnc.org.uk/. Accessed 27 Oct 2011.
20. Jackson D, et al. Support for carers particularly those with multiple caring roles. Research Initiative for Long Term Neurological Conditions website. [Internet] 2011. Available from: http://www.ltnc.org.uk/. Accessed 27 Oct 2011.
21. A Framework of National Occupational Standards to support common core competences and principles for health and social care workers working with adults at the end of life. Leicester: National End of Life Care Programme/Department of Health/Skills for Care/Skills for Health; 2010.
22. The LTNC Reference Dataset. The Information Centre for Health and Social Care website. [Internet] 2010. Available from: http://www.ic.nhs.uk/webfiles/Services/Datasets/LTNC/LTNC%20Data%20Requirements%20v1.0.pdf. Accessed 27 Oct 2011.

Chapter 11
End of Life Care in Progressive Neurological Disease: Australia

Susan Mathers

Abstract People with a progressive neurological disease can benefit from an integrated model of care which addresses their health and disability care needs over the course of their illness, and helps them to plan for the end of life. Australians enjoy a modern, mandated health and social welfare system, but a coordinated approach to chronic disease management is yet to be fully realised. This article reviews Australian health and disability service arrangements for chronic neurological disease, including some of the problems that arise from dichotomous governance and funding responsibilities in a federal system. Increasing use of E-technology should foster better communication and more effective teamwork in the future. By reducing the need for travel, E-health will also provide greater equity of access to specialist services and education.

Keywords Disability • Chronic • Neurological • Multidisciplinary • Australia

To be having a debate about how to provide the best model of care to people with progressive neurological diseases is the mark of a prosperous society. In many developing countries, citizens who are so afflicted struggle to see any doctor, let alone a neurologist as part of a multidisciplinary team with state-subsidized health care and disability support services. That Australians enjoy all of these components of a modern, mandated health and welfare system is one of the blessings of a stable democracy and an educated population. Yet, despite the billions of dollars spent on health and disability care each year, the system never seems so efficient, so uncontroversial, or so equitable when viewed from within. The reasons for this can be found in the makeup of Australian society, the size and settlement of this continent, and the history of social policy development. By examining these three areas—the people, the geography, and the system—we can identify the strengths and shortcomings of the delivery of health and disability services to people with

S. Mathers, MB ChB, MRCP (UK), FRACP
Neurology Unit, Calvary Health Care Bethlehem,
476 Kooyong Road, Caulfield, Melbourne, VIC 3121, Australia
e-mail: smathers@bethlehem.org.au

D. Oliver (ed.), *End of Life Care in Neurological Disease*,
DOI 10.1007/978-0-85729-682-5_11, © Springer-Verlag London 2013

chronic neurological conditions. This narrative aims to highlight areas where reforms could redirect the energies and resources which are our commonwealth.

The People

Like many New World countries with First World economies, Australia's prime disparity of health and well-being is between its indigenous and nonindigenous citizens. Aboriginal and Torres Strait Islander people make up 2.5 % of the Australian population but up to a quarter of the population in some regions. Life expectancy of indigenous people falls some 10 years short of the national averages. Standard mortality ratios for indigenous groups between 2004 and 2008 were 2–4 times the expected rate, and suicides were 3–5 times higher. The main causes of death are cardiovascular disease, trauma, malignancy, and diabetes [1]. Aboriginal people are known to carry a low genetic susceptibility to multiple sclerosis [2], the main cause of nontraumatic chronic neurological disability in young people in our society, but the prevalence of neurodegenerative conditions is not accurately known.

European settlement of Australia began in 1788, when Britain transported convicts to the colony that had been named New South Wales 18 years earlier by the explorer Captain James Cook. The multiple waves of migration which followed have helped swell the population to 22 million people from some 200 different countries. Since the end of transportation, people have come to Australia for social and economic reasons and as refugees in search of asylum. Britain remains the commonest country of origin for those born overseas, but since the 1970s, Australia has become an increasingly diverse social mix and one of the most successful multicultural societies. With this diversity of race, culture, language, and religion, it would therefore be surprising if a "one-size-fits-all" approach to health care was successful, especially in the contentious areas of illness behavior, the autonomy of the individual, and decisions around care at the end of life.

End of life care for people with neurological conditions cannot be dissociated from the quality and aims of their care throughout the often long course of their illness. Because patterns of neurological disability can be foreseen, it is the planning of therapeutic and social interventions along the way which affords some choice around how and where the end of life can be managed. The benefits of professional foresight, the timely anticipation of problems, and the exercise of this choice can all be maximized by a "long-term" model of care, not restricted to the "end of life" period alone. Physical disability and disturbances of cognition, behavior, and mood all play major roles in the dependency of the individual. In many cases, social and financial marginalization is the result. Impaired judgment often compromises decision making, and this may go unrecognized by family, carers, and health professionals. These effects are much more burdensome in neurological patients than in most other chronic disease groups and are more likely to lead to carer stress, crisis management, or default admission to hospital or residential care.

Palliative Care Australia (PCA) estimates that carers provide an estimated 76 % of all services to people needing care and support [3] and that "Many carers are not equipped with adequate support, training and resources to enable them to carry out their end of life care responsibilities effectively." [4] In an Australian survey, carers reported the lowest level of well-being of any population group [5]. The Productivity Commission (2011) warns that demographic change and the anticipated decline in the availability of informal care are expected to place further pressure on the existing system over the coming decades [6].

Euthanasia is not legal in Australia. Most states have strong medical treatment legislation that codifies patient autonomy, and advance care planning is endorsed by governments and is being increasingly adopted throughout all of the states and territories [7].

The Geography

In the minds of many people who have never visited Australia are images of its wide open spaces, the unusual fauna, and an outdoor lifestyle. In fact, Australia is, and has been from the time of European colonization, an urban nation. Most people live in the narrow, fertile southern and eastern coastal rim of the continent. Eight capital cities and a handful of large regional towns contain 85 % of its population. Tertiary health care services are strongly focused in the capital cities. Telecommunications have sustained rural and remote communities from the early days of the telegraph, allaying isolation and providing schooling for children and access to emergency relief (Flying Doctor Services). But rural and remote residents who require specialist or chronic treatment often face long periods removed from their homes and local communities. The distances these patients need to travel to their nearest city can be prohibitive for very disabled or terminally ill people. Victoria, for example, is one of the smallest states with a population of around five million people living in an area greater than the whole of the United Kingdom. Our one motor neuron disease (MND) clinic in Melbourne sees people from all over Victoria and the borders of adjacent states. Approximately 30 % of the people in Victoria with MND live outside greater metropolitan Melbourne, necessitating long periods of travel to attend clinics.

The System

It is self-evident that people living with a progressive neurological disease require a flexible, evolving range of resources if important goals are to be met as the disability increases. These include providing adequate support to their informal carers, as well as creating the circumstances which will allow them to remain in the residence of their choice, and if possible to die there. Ideal interprofessional health care should draw from expertise in neurology, rehabilitation, and palliative disciplines [8]. The provision of social and community services and financial support needs to match the trajectory of the underlying illness, anticipating health care changes and meeting the same milestones and contingencies in the life of that person. Yet, in Australia, governance and funding of health care and disability support services rest with two separate government departments, and at two different levels of government—state and federal. Eligibility for certain services varies with age (above and below 65 years) and with the cause of the disability; provisions are usually not translational across state boundaries. In their recent report, "Disability Care and Support," July 2011, the Australian Productivity Commission stated:

> The Australian Government is committed to developing a National Disability Strategy to enhance the quality of life and increase economic and social participation for people with disability and their carers..............The current disability support system is underfunded, unfair, fragmented, and inefficient, and gives people with a disability little choice and no certainty of access to appropriate supports [6].

Many of these dichotomies have occurred for historical and political reasons. There are, within Australian society, streams of national philosophy and ideology that favor, on the one hand, a centrally administrated health service based on equity and public funding, and on the other hand, a freedom to engage health service providers in commercial, fee-for-service arrangements. Although long-running political debates were eventually settled in the 1990s in favor of a universal public health system (Medicare), there still exists a strong private insurance sector which does attract some public funding and which operates in parallel to public hospitals to deliver some of the same services. A great deal of outpatient primary and specialist medical care and diagnostic services is performed within a private framework, though substantially subsidized by Medicare. The checks and balances of the democratic process have shaped policy development and delivered a degree of choice to most Australians. Yet, ironically, it is this dichotomous arrangement between health and disability services, private and public medicine and state versus federal responsibilities which lies at the heart of the difficulty in delivering an integrated, continuous model of care to people with chronic illness [9].

Although models of chronic disease management and patient-centered care are widely endorsed [8–10], actual system reform is slow, with government and media focused on the unrelenting pressure of overburdened emergency departments and protracted waiting lists within the acute system. Better chronic disease management could, of course, mitigate at least some of these burdens.

> There is a need for system redesign to meet the needs of individuals with chronic disease. New models of chronic disease care include team-based paradigms that focus on continuous and patient-centred care. In such models the roles of providers and patients must change......Effective components of these models include self-management support, use of clinical information systems, decision support and multidisciplinary teamwork [10].

The Strategic Plan 2008–2011 of Palliative Care Australia [11] promotes "quality care at the end of life for all," which "must be available regardless of diagnosis or prognosis." They define the "end of life" as that part lived with and impaired by an eventually fatal condition, where death in the foreseeable future would not be a surprise. They recommend strong networks of specialist and generalist providers working together.

In reality, this collaborative model has not, for a number of reasons, yet been fully realized. There is a need to improve the competency of all health professionals in end of life care. Much of the current palliative care resource is still focused on care of people dying of malignancy and even then during the last few weeks of life. Affording good palliative care to people dying of nonmalignant, including neurological, conditions is a work in progress. Care of catastrophic stroke in the acute sector and MND in the chronic sector are both perhaps at the vanguard of changing practice.

There is increasing involvement of palliative care specialists in the care of people dying in acute hospitals, especially in the tertiary hospitals with a strong palliative care presence. Pathways for improving the care of the dying [12] are providing better education of junior staff to recognize when patients are transitioning to the dying phase of their illness and helping all staff to realize the aims of good end of life care for patients and their families. As in many other countries, specialist multidisciplinary clinics for the care of people with MND have developed in Australia. Most have grown out of neurological practice, but some have their foundations in palliative care or rehabilitation medicine. All try to incorporate the many other areas of expertise that people with MND require. Inadequate funding of allied health professional support for these services is one of the main brakes on extending this successful model of care to more people with progressive neurological diseases. It is also fair to say that medical specialists (and doctors generally) have yet to fully embrace collaborative care or perhaps are not yet able to articulate their role within a collaborative care model. As recently as January 2010, the Royal Australasian College of Physicians wrote in a submission to the National Health and Medical Research Council on the "Ethical Issues Involved in the Transition to Palliation and End of Life Care for People with Chronic Conditions." [13]

> The Discussion Paper appears to assume that all patients should have access to specialised palliative care services during the transition to the terminal phase of their illness. An important question not addressed, is whether patients are best served by ongoing care from their usual doctors, with whom they may have built a relationship over many years, versus a change to other health professionals with specialised skills in palliative care, but who often are less skilled in the treatment of the underlying chronic disease...........The Discussion Paper alludes to the possibility of shared care between the active carers and those providing palliative care. This has the possibility to introduce confusion for patients and doctors.

A great deal of work still needs to be done on how we train doctors to hold differing roles—the role we are all most comfortable with in the dedicated doctor-patient relationship and the role within the multidisciplinary team. Often within the wider team, the role is of the leader and the chief negotiator for that team. As already argued, the team needs to include all of the people the patient elects to be part of their care—the so-called team without walls [14].

Outside the main hospital system, the makeup of community palliative care teams is quite variable. Most have a strong nursing focus, and most provide psychosocial support, some alternative therapies and volunteer services. The amount of dedicated palliative medicine specialist support within the team varies from one service to another but is often quite limited. Australia has about half the palliative medicine specialists it needs [15]. Many services rely on the general practitioner to provide medical input to the palliative management of the patient. With fewer GPs providing home visits or after-hours care, this responsibility can then fall to locum services.

Specialist neurological input to the patient's care at the end of life is often lost, unless these communication pathways have been predetermined by the multidisciplinary team. There are significant workforce shortages in rural areas across all disciplines.

The Future

The Australian system is in the early stages of health service and social care reform to address the future needs of an aging society and an increasing chronic disease burden. The current Labor Australian Government has given in-principle support for a National Disability Insurance Scheme. It is likely to take nearly a decade to fully implement. The National Health and Hospitals Reform Commission report (2009); "A Healthier Future For All Australians' picks up on the need to encourage 'better continuity and coordinated care for people with more complex health problems—including people with chronic diseases and disabilities…that can help coordinate, guide and navigate access to the right range of multidisciplinary health service providers…" and to promote the "better use of specialists in the community, recognising the central role of specialists to the shared management of care for patients with complex and chronic health needs." [9] The national Neurological Alliance and the author have reinforced the desirability of long-term models of care and a "specialist care coordinator" role to assist people with progressive neurological conditions to negotiate their care and join up their service providers [16–18].

The Australian government is currently commissioning a national broadband scheme, deploying a high-speed fiber network to 93 % of Australian homes, schools, and businesses with wireless or satellite connections for others [19]. This expensive and for some, controversial, public infrastructure spending will provide the connectivity that is required to reform the model of care for people living with and dying from progressive neurological diseases. Telehealth, case conferencing, peer support, education, and shared electronic records will all be enabled across the whole country. From July 2011, Medicare will fund telehealth consultations between specialists and GPs or nurses supporting patients in remote, regional, and outer metropolitan Australia [20].

Nurse practitioners have an emerging role in Australia, and there is a growing emphasis on training more general physicians to work outside metropolitan areas. New medical schools aim to draft students from regional and rural areas, and there are incentive schemes to attract health professionals to work in parts of Australia where there are workforce shortages. Access to good primary health care is increasingly important as people become more disabled and progress to the terminal phase of their illness. Beginning in 2011, the federal government is funding the development of a national network of primary health care organizations (Medicare Locals) to support the integration of health care, to improve the delivery of primary care services at a local level, and to improve access to allied health professionals and after-hours care [21].

To be efficient, equitable, and responsive, the new model must draw on the skills of a diverse workforce, both in the community and in the clinic. It aims to deliver better care to people closer to their home and to reduce demand on the acute health care sector. Recognizing that not all of the needs of people with life-limiting and disabling disease can be met by a clinical model of care alone, the model needs to find the required synergy between clinical and psychosocial supports. The greatest challenge to how we train and deploy our future workforce will be fostering effective teamwork. E-technology promises to provide the network for such teamwork across this continent.

References

1. Australian Bureau of Statistics. Australian government. http://www.abs.gov.au. Accessed 31 Aug 2011.
2. Roberts-Thomson PJ, Roberts-Thomson RA, Nikoloutsopoulos T, Gillis D. Immune dysfunction in Australian aborigines. Asian Pac J Allergy Immunol. 2005;23(4):235–44.
3. Palliative Care Australia (PCA). The hardest thing we have ever done – the social impact of caring for terminally ill people in Australia 2004: full report of the national inquiry into the social impact of caring for terminally ill Australians, PCA, Canberra, 2004.
4. Palliative Care Australia. Position statement. Carers and end of life. http://www.palliativecare. org.au. Accessed 28 Aug 2011.
5. Cummins RA, Hughes J, Tomyn A, Gibson A, Woerner J, Lai L. Australian Unity Wellbeing Index, Survey 17.1, Oct 2007. The wellbeing of Australians – carer health and wellbeing. Deakin University, Australian Unity Ltd and Carers Australia, Melbourne. 2007. http://www. deakin.edu.au/research/acqol/index_wellbeing/index.htm. Accessed 28 Aug 2011.
6. Australian Government. Productivity commission inquiry report – disability care and support. 2011. http://www.pc.gov.au. Accessed 29 Aug 2011.
7. Respecting Patient Choices, Advanced Care Planning. Project funded under the National Palliative Care Program, supported by the Australian Government and the Victorian Department of Health. http://www.respectingpatientchoices.org.au. Accessed 31 Aug 2011.
8. Royal College of Physicians UK. National Guidelines No. 10 Long-term neurological conditions: management at the interface between neurology, rehabilitation and palliative care. 2008.
9. National Health and Hospitals Reform Commission. A healthier future for all Australians – final report. 2009. http://www.yourhealth.gov.au. Accessed 5 Sept 2011.
10. Brand C, Greenberg P, Sargious P. Chronic disease management: time for consultant physicians to take more leadership in system redesign. Intern Med J. 2007;37(9):653–9.
11. Palliative Care Australia. Strategic plan 2008–2011. http://www.palliativecare.org.au. Accessed 17 Aug 2011.
12. Jackson K, Mooney C, Campbell D. The development and implementation of the pathway for improving the care of the dying in general medical wards. Intern Med J. 2009;39(10):695–9.
13. Submission to the National Health and Medical Research Council on the Ethical Issues Involved in the Transitions to Palliation and End of Life Care for People with Chronic Conditions on behalf of The Royal Australasian College of Physicians. 2010. http://www.racp. edu.au. Accessed 4 Sept 2011.
14. Steel J, Burnham R. Teams without walls: enabling partnerships between generalists and specialists. Clin Med. 2009;9(1):74–5.
15. Palliative Care Australia – Position Statement. Workforce for quality care at the end of life. http://www.palliativecare.org.au. Accessed 17 Aug 2011.

16. Neurological Alliance Australia. Submission to the productivity commission's inquiry into disability care and support. 2010. http://www.pc.gov.au/_data/assets/pdf_file/0017/102752/sub0521.pdf. Accessed 3 Sept 2011.
17. Mathers S. Submission to the productivity commission's inquiry into disability care and support. Continuous care for people with a progressive neurological disability. 2010. Submission No. 436.
18. MS Australia (ACT,NSW,Vic) and Calvary Health Care Bethlehem. The continuous care pilot – final report. 2010. http://www.mssociety.org.au/documents/CCCPilot/TOTAL-combined-CCP-REPORT-FINAL.pdf. Accessed on 3 Sept 2011.
19. Australian Government. National broadband network. http://www.nbn.gov.au. Accessed on 3 Sept 2011.
20. Australian Government. Connecting health services with the future: modernising medicare by providing rebates for on-line consultations. 2011. http://www.mbsonline.gov.au/telehealth. Accessed 3 Sept 2011.
21. Australian Government. Department of health and ageing. National health reform-medicare locals. http://www.yourhealth.gov.au/internet/yourhealth/publishing.nsf/content/medilocals-lp-1. Accessed 3 Sept 2011.

Chapter 12
International Aspects of Care: Europe

Simone Veronese

Abstract Across Europe there is much variation in both the neurology and palliative care services provided for people with progressive neurological disease.
However there is increasing interest and collaboration in some areas. These initiatives are being developed across Europe, with improvement in the end of life care
for patients and families.

Keywords Development of services • Variation • Research • International
perspective • Tertiary centers

Introduction

Europe can be defined from different perspectives: in the World Health Organization
(WHO) it is represented by 53 countries [1], at the Council of Europe is represented
by 47 nations [2], whereas the European Union comprises of 27 independent states
[3]. This variation shows how difficult it is to properly define Europe. Moreover, the
health-care systems vary greatly over the whole of Europe, with differences in availability, funding, and development of palliative and end of life programmes [4].

There are also differences as to how neurology is seen across Europe. In many
countries neurology services are closely involved in the care of people with brain
tumours – whereas in others, this care is coordinated by oncology services. There
are similar variations in services for people with dementia – who are seen as part of
psychiatric or psychogeriatric services in some areas. However, despite these variations, there are numerous initiatives developing in many countries related to the end
of life care for people dying of neurological conditions [5].

Since St Christopher's Hospice was opened in 1967 in the UK, and the new era
of palliative care started, the involvement in the care of people with neurological

S. Veronese
Department of Palliative Care, FARO Foundation,
Turin, Italy
e-mail: simone.veronese@fondazionefaro.it

D. Oliver (ed.), *End of Life Care in Neurological Disease*,
DOI 10.1007/978-0-85729-682-5_12, © Springer-Verlag London 2013

disease has increased. Dame Cicely Saunders, founder of St. Christopher's Hospice and pioneer of modern palliative care, wrote in 1981:

> Our Lady's Hospice in Dublin (1879) and St Joseph's Hospice in London (1905) both included patients with long-term illness in their wards and St Christopher's Hospice (1967) followed this tradition and opened with at least 10 % of its ward beds for patients with advanced neurological illnesses. The need of patients with motor neurone disease continues and their care has been integrate into the life of the hospice [6].

More recently the first specialist book describing the role of palliative care in neurology has been published and the majority of the editors are European, underlying the importance of their role in these disciplines [7]. There is also a taskforce of the European Association for Palliative Care looking at developing guidelines on neurological palliative care and the curriculum for training both palliative care and neurology professionals.

The European initiatives regarding end of life care for amyotrophic lateral sclerosis (ALS or motor neurone disease), multiple sclerosis (MS), and Parkinson's disease will be reviewed, and a snapshot of the Italian experience will be presented as an example.

Amyotrophic Lateral Sclerosis (ALS)

ALS is the neurological disease with the most settled relationship with palliative care because of the relentless progression of its nature leading to death in 2–4 years [8]. The first evidence of the involvement of palliative care was in the UK, and again is reported by Dame Cicely Saunders in a letter that she wrote in 1990 to Dr. Mary Eleanor Toms stating that at St Christopher they had been caring for patients in terminal stages of motor neuron disease since the opening of the hospice, and that their first patient had been admitted in 1967 [9].

Since then there have been many developments. In 1985 a British group published a paper stating that even in the most severe forms of ALS, the symptoms and disabilities may be relieved applying the principles of management of all progressive incurable diseases and the quality of life for patients may be improved even in the terminal stages, in home or hospice [10]. In 1992 the first data describing the role of hospice care in ALS were disclosed in the UK showing the efficacy of opioids in the treatment of symptoms like pain and breathlessness and the appropriateness of the admissions [11].

The interest for end of life care for ALS spread throughout Europe, and international collaborations started among different groups involved in palliative care. A multicentre study showed that good palliative care can allow a peaceful death process in ALS, confirming the safety of opioid and benzodiazepine medications and providing indications for the use of PEG and home mechanical ventilation [12].

After the publication of the American Academy of Neurologists of the first evidence-based guidelines for the treatment of ALS patients [13], recommendations were published in Germany for the most important symptoms arising in the end stage of neurological diseases with a particular focus on ALS. These recommendations include treatment of dyspnoea, death rattle, restlessness, pain, thirst, and depression [14].

Italian and Irish neurologists have shown the importance of multidisciplinary care in ALS showing how the impact of such complex disorder on patients and carers can be alleviated by an integrated approach [15, 16]. These multidisciplinary ALS clinics have developed in many areas and provide specialist care. However, many people with ALS are not seen by specialist services and may remain within general medical or rehabilitation services. The provision of clinics and specialist knowledge and provision of specialist interventions, such as gastrostomy placement, respiratory support using noninvasive ventilation, and involvement in trials of new potential medication, are very variable across the nations of Europe.

Multiple Sclerosis

In Europe there are numerous initiatives toward better understanding the needs of patients affected by advanced MS and their informal carers, and there is the high prevalence of this disorder in northern Europe countries [16]. A German group showed how professionals involved in the care of MS patients felt the key points in the improvement of the quality of life in this condition are the support from family and friends, the need for managing everyday life, the role of good health-care services, and the desire to maintain biographical continuity [17]. This is strongly consistent with previous qualitative studies in the UK that suggested that even patients who have had MS for many years and are now severely affected, continue to experience loss and change – and these studies recommend that attention be given to emotional support, physical issues, independence, and relationships [18].

A needs assessment conducted at the King's College of Hospital, London showed that many symptoms in people severely affected by MS are as highly prevalent and severe as those experienced by patients with advanced cancer and that increased disability is associated with increased severity for some symptoms [19]. All the cited researchers conclude their papers stating that the skills of palliative can care teams would be of help to MS patients with severe disability and their family carers.

The same group evaluated the involvement of palliative care in advanced MS patients in the southeast of London with a pilot RCT. The results show that the involvement with the palliative care service appeared to positively affect nausea and sleeping problems to some degree, with the effect strongest after initial contact with the clinical service. It also seemed to have a positive impact on informal carer well-being. User satisfaction with the service was high among MS patients, carers, and especially other health-care professionals. Availability of time, symptom management, end of life decision making and liaison appear to be important components of the service. Involvement with the palliative care service did not shorten life in patients severely affected by MS [20]. This short-term palliative care input has also showed to be cost-effective [21].

Parkinson's Disease and Movement Disorders

Movement disorders are a group of neurodegenerative conditions represented by the Parkinson's disease (PD) and by the atypical parkinsonian syndromes, such as multiple system atrophy (MSA) and progressive supranuclear palsy (PSP). Movement disorders traditionally were not considered as requiring palliative care, and there is limited information on the involvement of palliative care services in these conditions. However, in Europe there are several groups that provide care, and research has been undertaken on the relevance to the provision of palliative care. In the UK the quality of life and symptom prevalence have been explored in depth, providing new data about these issues, showing that pain is both prevalent, severe, and multifactorial in PD. It has also suggested that improving quality of life in PD should focus not only on physical but also psychosocial issues and that symptoms and psychosocial problems may be improved by input from a palliative care team [22–24].

European Initiatives

The European Association for Palliative Care (EAPC) constituted a taskforce for neurology that is now chaired by Dr David Oliver, a palliative care specialist from the UK well known for his studies and care in ALS. The taskforce is now producing the first guidelines on the topic of palliative and end of life care in neurology [25].

The National End of Life Care Programme in the UK recently published a document aiming to improve the end of life care in neurological diseases [26]. This report lists the challenges due to the particular issues of neurological conditions, provides indicators and triggers that help identify the end of life phase, and suggests when to start palliative care interventions and the involvement of palliative care services.

The Italian Experience

In Italy, palliative care has recently been regulated by a national law (Law 38/15th March 2010) named "Dispositions to guarantee the access to Palliative Care and Pain Therapy" [27]. This official document defines palliative care as "a complex of interventions for both patients and their families, aimed at the total and active care of those persons affected by progressive and relentless conditions, no longer responsive to specific treatments." The user of palliative care is defined as "a person affected by a chronic and progressive condition for which no curative therapies exist, or if exist are inadequate or inefficacious to stabilize the disease or to prolong significantly his or her life span."

According to this definition, a large number of potential users should receive palliative care in Italy. Until now, only a minority of patients dying for cancer can access palliative care, and the provision of these services for patients affected by nonmalignant conditions is rare and limited to occasional local initiatives.

Within the National Society of Neurology (SIN), a taskforce named "Group for the study of the Bioethics and Palliative Care" started in 2000, involving neurologists, palliative care physicians, rehabilitation specialists, and other nonmedical professionals. Its main objectives are the analysis of bioethical issues relevant for neurology, promotion of research of palliative care in neurology, and education of professionals involved in this field [28].

Many documents relevant to these themes have been published by this group, including a general paper discussing the involvement palliative care in neurology [29, 30], palliative sedation in neurology [31], advance directives [32], discontinuation of life-support measures in patients in a permanent vegetative state [33], and end of life treatments in the dementia patient [34].

Patients with ALS are more likely to receive in palliative care in Italy. Several palliative care units do deliver their services to patients affected by ALS, even though a small minority of patients dying of ALS receive hospice care in Italy. Barriers to the access to palliative care services are usually represented by the lack of knowledge of professionals about the disease itself, lack of networking among neurological centers and hospices, difficulties in predicting the timing of referrals, and, unfortunately, fear of opioids in the management of breathlessness and other symptoms. The option of palliative care is rarely suggested by neurologists to patients and their families, and very few specialists feel comfortable in discussing the possibility of palliative care and death and dying with patients.

In Italy, there are also tertiary centres totally committed to the care and research in ALS. The PARALS register is a population-based register and is run within Piedmonte, and it is linked to the CRESLA that is the regional expert center for ALS [35]. Palliative and hospice care is now available for patients living in this area since some PCU were actively involved in the CRESLA. Research has also started in this area. FARO Foundation, a charity providing specialist palliative care in Turin City and its province, has founded and started a process of design and assessment of a new SPCS for people severely affected by neurodegenerative conditions. This followed a study in which a randomized and controlled trial between a group of patients who received SPCS immediately and a control group who had a wait of 16 weeks showed a significant improvement in patients' individual quality of life and symptoms control. A new service is now fully operative for patients with ALS and this will be extended to patients multiple sclerosis and Parkinson's disease in 2012/3. [36].

Conclusion

Across Europe, there is increasing involvement of palliative care services with people with advanced neurological disease, and there are areas of excellence. However, overall, patients rarely receive the help they may need, and there is a need for further development of services and change in attitudes of patients, families, and professionals.

References

1. WHO. World Health Organisation Regional Office for Europe website. World Health Organisation; 2012 [cited Feb 8 2012]. Available from: http://www.euro.who.int/en/where-we-work.
2. Europe Co. The Council of Europe website. 2012 [cited Feb 1 2012]. Available from: http://www.coe.int/lportal/web/coe-portal.
3. EUROPA.EU. The European Union Portal. 2012 [cited Feb 1 2012]. Available from: http://europa.eu/about-eu/countries/index_it.htm.
4. De Conno F, Blumhuber H, Rocafort J. The development of palliative medicine in Europe. In: Bruera E, Higginson I, Ripamonti C, Von Gunten C, editors. Textbook of palliative medicine. 1st ed. London: Hodder Arnold; 2009. p. 12–21.
5. Borasio GD, Voltz R. Palliative care in neurology. J Palliat Care. 2005;21(3):188–9.
6. Saunders C, Walsh D, Smith M. Hospice care in motor neurone disease. In: Saunders C, Summers D, Teller N, editors. Hospice: the living idea. London: Edward Arnold; 1981. p. 126–55.
7. Voltz R, Bernat JL, Borasio GD, Maddocks I, Oliver D, Portenoy RK. (editors). Palliative care in neurology Oxford: Oxford University Press; 2004.
8. Ringel SP, Murphy JR, Alderson MK, Bryan W, England JD, Miller RG, et al. The natural history of amyotrophic lateral sclerosis. Neurology. 1993;43(7):1316–22.
9. Clark D. Cicely Saunders. Founder of the hospice movement. Selected letters 1959–1999. Oxford: Oxford University Press; 2002.
10. Norris FH, Smith RA, Denys EH. Motor neurone disease: towards better care. Br Med J (Clin Res Ed). 1985;291(6490):259–62.
11. O'Brien T, Kelly M, Saunders C. Motor neurone disease: a hospice perspective. BMJ. 1992;304(6825):471–3.
12. Neudert C, Oliver D, Wasner M, Borasio GD. The course of the terminal phase in patients with amyotrophic lateral sclerosis. J Neurol. 2001;248(7):612–6.
13. Miller RG, Rosenberg JA, Gelinas DF, Mitsumoto H, Newman D, Sufit R, et al. Practice parameter: the care of the patient with amyotrophic lateral sclerosis (an evidence-based review): report of the Quality Standards Subcommittee of the American Academy of Neurology: ALS Practice Parameters Task Force. Neurology. 1999;52(7):1311–23.
14. Voltz R, Borasio GD. Palliative therapy in the terminal stage of neurological disease. J Neurol. 1997;244 Suppl 4:S2–10.
15. Chio A, Bottacchi E, Buffa C, Mutani R, Mora G. Positive effects of tertiary centres for amyotrophic lateral sclerosis on outcome and use of hospital facilities. J Neurol Neurosurg Psychiatry. 2006;77(8):948–50.
16. Traynor BJ, Alexander M, Corr B, Frost E, Hardiman O. Effects of a multidisciplinary ALS clinic on survival. J Neurol Neurosurg Psychiatry. 2003;74:1258–61.
17. Golla H, Galushko M, Pfaff H, Voltz R. Unmet needs of severely affected multiple sclerosis patients: the health professionals' view. Palliat Med. 2011;26(2):139–51.
18. Edmonds P, Vivat B, Burman R, Silber E, Higginson IJ. Loss and change: experiences of people severely affected by multiple sclerosis. Palliat Med. 2007;21(2):101–7.
19. Higginson IJ, Hart S, Silber E, Burman R, Edmonds P. Symptom prevalence and severity in people severely affected by multiple sclerosis. J Palliat Care. 2006;22(3):158–65.
20. Edmonds P, Hart S, Wei G, Vivat B, Burman R, Silber E. Palliative care for people severely affected by multiple sclerosis: evaluation of a novel palliative care service. Mult Scler. 2010;16(5):627–36.
21. Higginson IJ, McCrone P, Hart SR, Burman R, Silber E, Edmonds PM. Is short-term palliative care cost-effective in multiple sclerosis? A randomized phase II trial. J Pain Symptom Manage. 2009;38(6):816–26.
22. Lee MA, Walker RW, Hildreth TJ, Prentice WM. A survey of pain in idiopathic Parkinson's disease. J Pain Symptom Manage. 2006;32(5):462–9.

23. Lee MA, Walker RW, Hildreth AJ, Prentice WM. Individualized assessment of quality of life in idiopathic Parkinson's disease. Mov Disord. 2006;21(11):1929–34.
24. Lee MA, Prentice WM, Hildreth AJ, Walker RW. Measuring symptom load in Idiopathic Parkinson's disease. Parkinsonism Relat Disord. 2007;13(5):284–9.
25. EAPC. People with neurological disease. 2012 [cited Feb 8 2012]. Available from: http://www.eapcnet.eu/Themes/Specificgroups/Peoplewithneurologicaldisease/Guidelinescurriculumtaskforce.aspx.
26. NHS. Improving end of life care in neurological disease. A framework for implementation. 2010 [cited Feb 8 2012]. Available from: http://www.endoflifecareforadults.nhs.uk/publications/end-of-life-care-in-long-term-neurological-conditions-a-framework.
27. Law 38,15.3.10. Republic of Italy: Disposizioni per garantire l'accesso alle cure palliative ed alla terapia del dolore. 2010. Access at: http://www.parlamento.it/parlam/leggi/10038l.htm.
28. Defanti CA. Study Group of Bioethics and Palliative Care in Neurology: program document. Neurol Sci. 2000;21(5):261–71.
29. Causarano R. Le cure palliative in neurologia: come, dove e quando. Neurol Sci. 2005;26:S127–31.
30. Defanti CA. Come muore il malato neurologico? Neurol Sci. 2005;26:S109–13.
31. Bonito V, Caraceni A, Borghi L, Marcello N, Mori M, Porteri C, et al. The clinical and ethical appropriateness of sedation in palliative neurological treatments. Neurol Sci. 2005;26(5):370–85.
32. Bonito V. Le dichiarazione anticipate in neurologia. Neurol Sci. 2005;26:S121–6.
33. Bonito V, Primavera A, Borghi L, Mori M, Defanti CA. The discontinuation of life support measures in patients in a permanent vegetative state. Neurol Sci. 2002;23(3):131–9.
34. Congedo M, Causarano RI, Alberti F, Bonito V, Borghi L, Colombi L, et al. Ethical issues in end of life treatments for patients with dementia. Eur J Neurol. 2010;17(6):774–9.
35. Chio A, Mora G, Leone M, Mazzini L, Cocito D, Giordana MT, et al. Early symptom progression rate is related to ALS outcome: a prospective population-based study. Neurology. 2002;59(1):99–103.
36. Veronese S, Oliver D, editors. Developing and evaluating a specialist palliative care service for people with neurodegenerative disorders. An application of the MRC framework for the design and the evaluation of complex interventions. In: 12th conference of the European Association for Palliative Care, Lisbon, 2011.

Chapter 13
International Aspects of Care: Africa

Liz Gwyther

Abstract Palliative care services in Africa have been involved in the care of people with motor neuron disease for many years and the aim has been to work in a collaborative way with all services, to improve quality of care for patients and their families. Due to the particular circumstances in Africa this has extended to involvement with the neurological complications of HIV infection and neurosurgical services, for people following head injury or surgery.

Keywords HIV infection • Progressive disease • Neurosurgery • Limited resources • WHO

Palliative care in Africa developed initially as a response to the needs of patients with advanced cancer as with many palliative care services. Hospice services in South Africa extended the reach of palliative care to patients with motor neuron disease and other progressive neurological disorders as patients with these conditions presented to hospice. The Motor Neurone Disease Association of South Africa has a strong service providing information, support, practical assistance, clinical care to patients, and support to family members [1].

Since the 1990s, palliative care in Africa has been increasingly involved in the care of patients with advanced HIV, and the picture of palliative care has changed. The palliative care response to needs of HIV patients means that the scope of palliative care has increased to include treatment support of patients on antiretroviral medication and nutritional support, addressing with varying degrees of success the economic challenges that face HIV-positive patients and their families. Many hospices have implemented "wellness programs" for HIV-positive patients whose condition has improved through access to antiretroviral treatment but who continue to need lifelong treatment support and psychosocial support [2].

L. Gwyther, MB ChB, FCFP, M.Sc. Pall Med
Hospice Palliative Care Association of South Africa,
Howard Place, 7450, Suite 11a, Lonsdale Building,
Lonsdale Way 38785, Pinelands, 7430, South Africa
e-mail: liz@hpca.co.za

D. Oliver (ed.), *End of Life Care in Neurological Disease*,
DOI 10.1007/978-0-85729-682-5_13, © Springer-Verlag London 2013

The World Health Organization states that palliative care is "applicable early in the course of illness," and the WHO definition of palliative care for children is that "it begins when the illness is diagnosed." Three palliative care services in Africa have made an effort to respond to the need for palliative care earlier in the course of the illness. Hospices are not able to take on the responsibility of all people requiring palliative care so it has become increasingly important to build the capacity of health care professionals in all fields to provide supportive and palliative care to patients earlier in the trajectory of the illness including recognition of the patient's palliative care needs.

Progressive Neurological Disorders

South Africa is the only country in Africa that has a registered Motor Neurone Disease Association (MNDA) and provides advice to families and clinicians in other African countries. The MNDA in South Africa reports that there are about 200 patients registered with the association. This is a fraction of the anticipated number of patients with MND in South Africa. If the prevalence of the illness is similar to that in Europe and North America, MNDA SA would anticipate 3,000 MND patients in the country. The association provides physical assistance, psychological counselling and support for patients and carers, and equipment loan. The MNDA of SA is affiliated with the Hospice Palliative Care Association of South Africa, and hospice staff work closely with MNDA staff and volunteers to provide care in the person's home.

International links are important in ensuring that advances in patient care can be implemented and in supporting the MNDA in South Africa. Patients are mostly cared for in their homes with admission to hospice or frail care (care home) settings for short periods or for terminal care.

Symptom management for patients requires a good assessment and individualized management, and the most important aspect of care for people with MND is good communication to patient and family carers so that they can understand the progression of the illness and the assistance that is available or that can be provided by carers at home. The biggest challenge to care is the difficulty patients and families have in adjusting to the diagnosis and the disease progression. Sometimes, this difficulty in adjustment to the realities of MND means that people do not receive the care that would be most helpful.

Areas where palliative care services may be able to provide particular help and advice include:

- Symptom management: Progressive weakness is hard to adjust to, especially for people who have had a particularly physically active lifestyle. It is important to continue to exercise both for physical mobility and psychological well-being. Physiotherapy is important, and family members can be involved in providing home physiotherapy – both active and passive – with advice and instruction from a physiotherapist. Home aids are important, and the MNDA provides particular assistance with these. The challenge in rural South Africa and in other African countries is the competing priorities in health care that make provision of devices to assist with mobility rare.

- Pain may be experienced as a result of muscle spasm or muscle stiffness, and baclofen may be prescribed to relieve this symptom. For other causes of pain, appropriate assessment and management according to the WHO guidelines assists in pain control.
- Dyspnea: Low-dose morphine is used in reducing the sensation of dyspnea, and benzodiazepine assists in breaking the cycle of anxiety, dyspnea, and panic. The use of noninvasive ventilation is not common in the African setting but is used for people that can access this technology.
- Dysphagia: A dietitian's advice is a useful part of the multidisciplinary approach to care of the person with MND; family members are often very distressed by the patient being unable to swallow food offered to them, and sensitive counselling to discuss slow feeding, pureed food, cloths to deal with secretions, and drooling as well as food that cannot be swallowed is important in adjusting to living with MND. The insertion of PEG feeding tube is uncommon in Africa.
- Emotional liability and depression: This is another aspect of the illness that requires careful explanation and support as patients are particularly distressed when they feel that their emotions are out of control.

Palliative Care for Patients with Neurological Conditions Associated with HIV Infection

A significant proportion of patients cared for by hospices in Africa are HIV positive, and there are a number of neurological conditions that occur especially in patients with stage 3 and 4 HIV, involving further investigation and treatment as suggested by in the WHO definition of palliative care – "those investigations needed to better understand and manage distressing clinical complications." [3]

The human immunodeficiency virus (HIV) is a neurotrophic virus that infects the central and peripheral nervous system so that neurological symptoms are widely prevalent at all stages of HIV infection. It is estimated that 40–70 % of people infected with HIV develop neurological symptoms. In addition to the neurological disturbances caused by HIV infection, antiretroviral treatment can have significant neurological side effects. Highly active antiretroviral treatment has impacted significantly on life span and quality of life for HIV-positive patients, and the access to affordable medication has been instrumental in changing the prognosis for HIV patients [4]. It is of concern that not all African countries and not all HIV-positive patients have access to these critical medications. The recommendations for initiation on HAART include a CD4 count of <350 cells/µL. However, in many African countries, people still present late; in South Africa, the average CD4 count for initiation of HAART, as reported in 2011, was 170 cells/µL. Opportunistic infections and other complications may be less when people are initiated on HAART earlier in the course of the infection.

Opportunistic Infections

Meningitis is common in HIV infection, and it is important that patients with unexpected headache and fever have a lumbar puncture (LP) – provided there are no focal signs or papilledema. It is advised to measure cerebrospinal fluid (CSF) pressure when doing the LP as a raised CSF pressure is suggestive of cryptococcal meningitis. Common neurological infections include cryptococcal meningitis, tuberculous meningitis, meningovascular syphilis, pneumococcal meningitis, viral meningitis, and encephalitis. Treatment of the infective organism according to standard regimes is the cornerstone of managing neurological infections. Serial drainage of CSF has been used to control the headache of cryptococcal meningitis.

Parenchymal Brain Disease

HIV infection can result in the development of cognitive and behavioral changes which range from mild cognitive or motor deficit to HIV-associated dementia in advanced disease. The response to HAART is rapid and usually complete. In the early days of HIV management in South Africa, one of the conditions for receiving HIV was understanding the illness and treatment (termed treatment literacy) and normal cognition so that patients would understand and adhere to treatment [2]. This meant that patients with HIV-associated dementia could be excluded from receiving medication. However, with supervised administration of HAART until normal cognition was restored has allowed this group of patients to benefit from treatment.

Seizures

Seizures in HIV-positive patients may be caused by a space-occupying lesion (toxoplasmosis or tuberculoma), meningitis, and metabolic disturbances. Sometimes, a cause cannot be identified other than HIV infection. It is important to identify the cause and institute appropriate management.

Stroke

Infection with the human immunodeficiency virus contributes to an increased risk of stroke, and the age of stroke patients who are HIV positive is lower than non-HIV infected stroke patients. For example, a report on the register of stroke patients at

Groote Schuur Hospital in Cape Town showed that of 1,087 stoke patients registered between 2000 and 2006, "67 (6.2 %) were identified as HIV infected. The mean age of the HIV infected stroke patients was 33.4 years while the mean age of the patients not determined to be HIV infected was 64.0 years." [5]

HIV-Related Neuropathy

Neuropathic pain is common in HIV-positive patients. However, it is often underdiagnosed and undertreated. Hitchcock comments that a lack of awareness of the extent of the problem may contribute to this inadequate management. The peripheral sensory neuropathy usually presents with painful dysesthesia and numbness or other sensory dysfunction in a "glove and stocking" distribution. Most commonly, it is the feet and lower legs that are affected. The problem is exacerbated by some drug treatment particularly isoniazid used for TB prophylaxis and TB treatment and stavudine (d4T), didanosine (ddI), and zalcitabine (ddC). Alternate regimens are advised for patients with neuropathy, and the South African treatment guidelines no longer use these drugs first-line because of the side effects [4].

A thorough assessment of neuropathic pain is essential, including objective clinical tests such as tests of tactile, pinprick, and vibration sensation. Guidelines to manage HIV neuropathic pain include non-pharmacological measures – sleep hygiene and graded physical activity, physiotherapy to reduce myofascial components that can exacerbate neuropathic pain- and combination pharmacology of tramadol or opioid medication first-line for acute neuropathic pain and exacerbations of neuropathic pain combined with medication targeting pain pathways such as amitriptyline, gabapentin or pregabalin, and duloxetine or venlafaxine or carbamazepine. An adequate trial of one of these medications should be implemented and only changed if there is no adequate response in pain levels. This presupposes recording of pain levels at assessment and reassessment of pain.

Palliative Care in the Neurosurgical Setting

There are a number of countries in Africa where intentional and non-intentional injuries contribute significantly to the burden of disease and to mortality. For example, in South Africa, intentional injuries contributed to 2 % of deaths in 2008 (WHO) compared to 0.12 % of deaths in the UK (9.9 % in Zimbabwe, 2.7 % in Uganda, 2.1 % in Kenya) [6]. As a result, there are a significant number of head injuries and neurosurgical procedures carried out on people who have suffered these injuries. A nongovernmental organization ComaCARE has been established at Groote Schuur Hospital in Cape Town to influence care of patients who are comatose or recovering from head injuries and from surgery for brain tumors and to support their family members during this period [7]. ComaCARE has invited a palliative care physician and palliative care social worker to assist in support of staff of the neurosurgical unit and of ComaCARE. Palliative care training has been provided to the staff to provide guidance on care of the patient who is dying. One of the programs developed is the Comeback program to assist in rehabilitation of patients recovering from coma. There is also a need to counsel family members if life support is considered no longer appropriate and to provide bereavement care. This innovative practice may prove a model to implement improved care of coma patients in other African hospitals.

Conclusion

Resources for specialized neurological care are limited in Africa, and there are significant neurological conditions associated with infections and with injuries that require skills and attitudes of palliative care. It is important that palliative care clinicians work alongside neurologists and neurosurgeons to learn from each discipline with the aim of providing quality care to patients and family members. Hospice workers who do not have access to specialist advice in Africa continue to support patients and family members with compassion and care according to knowledge and principles of palliative care.

References

1. Motor neurone disease association of South Africa. Available at: http://www.alsmndalliance. org/. Accessed 1 Mar 2012.
2. Harding R, Gwyther L, Mwangi-Powell F. Treating HIV/AIDS patients until the end of life. J Acquir Immune Defic Syndr. 2007;44(3):364.
3. World Health Organization. Palliative care. 2002. Available at: www.who.int/cancer/palliative/ definition/en/. Accessed 14 Apr 2012.
4. HPCA Clinical Guidelines. 2006. Available at: http://www.hospicepalliativecaresa.co.za/pdf/ guidelinedocs/HPCAClinicalGuidelines.pdf. Accessed 1 Mar 2012.
5. Tipping B, de Villiers L, Wainwright H, Candy S, Bryer A. Stroke in patients with human immunodeficiency virus infection. J Neurol Neurosurg Psychiatry. 2007;78:1320–4.
6. WHO. Mortality and global burden disease. 2008. Available at: http://www.who.int/gho/mortality_burden_disease/global_burden_disease_death_estimates_sex_2008.xls. Accessed 29 Aug 2011.
7. ComaCARE. 2010. Available at: http://www.comacare.com/. Accessed 1 Mar 2012.

Chapter 14
Conclusion

David Oliver

Abstract The care of a person with progressive neurological disease is complex and requires a multidisciplinary approach. The challenge for all services is the identification of the person who is deteriorating and for whom the emphasis of care is changing. There is the need to increase the awareness and encourage an open approach of all professionals so that people at the end of life can receive the care they require. This may include changing attitudes and education of all involved - patients, their families and professionals.

Keywords End of life care • Identification • Multidsicplinary care • Education

The care of a person with progressive neurological disease is complex and requires the involvement of a wide multidisciplinary team and careful discussion and collaboration of all involved – health and social care professionals, patient, and family/carers. There is increasing awareness of the importance of end of life care and the need for changing priorities and management as a person deteriorates. The importance of end of life has been highlighted in the UK with the publication of the report "End of life care in long term neurological conditions – a framework for implementation" [1] and more widely in Europe with the European Association for Palliative Care taskforce on neurological palliative care [2]. However, there is still a need for further developments across the UK, Europe, and worldwide.

The crucial issue may be the recognition that a person is deteriorating and dying and the identification of patient and families for whom end of life care would be appropriate. This may be achieved through the development of triggers which allow professional carers to identify patients and thus ensure that they are then managed in the most appropriate way. In the UK, the National Institute for Clinical Excellence has led the way by incorporating consideration of end of life care in its guidelines.

D. Oliver, B.Sc., FRCP, FRCGP
Wisdom Hospice, High Bank,
Rochester, Kent, ME1 2NU, UK
e-mail: drdjoliver@googlemail.com

D. Oliver (ed.), *End of Life Care in Neurological Disease*,
DOI 10.1007/978-0-85729-682-5_14, © Springer-Verlag London 2013

For instance, in the guideline on noninvasive ventilation in motor neurone disease [3], it is suggested that discussion of palliative and end of life care is included in the discussion before and at the instigation of treatment. This enables patients and families to be aware of the options available to them and take the opportunity to undertake advance care planning for the future.

There are challenges for all involved. This includes all the various medical and social care teams that may be involved in the care of the person with a progressive neurological disease. For instance, neurology services need to become more aware of end of life care issues and to recognize patients whose condition may be changing. There is also a need of palliative care and end of life care specialist teams to become more aware of the specific needs and issues of people with neurological disease – including knowledge about the disease itself, the medication or interventions that may be helpful, and the use of medication at the end of life.

Throughout the discussions within this book, it is clear that an awareness and recognition of the end of life needs of people with neurological disease will result in a greater emphasis on quality of life, when making management decisions. This can be achieved through:

- Careful discussion of the person's needs and wishes
- Consideration and assessment of all the issues:

  - Physical
  - Psychological/emotional
  - Social
  - Spiritual

- Discussion of advance care planning
- Involvement and collaboration with other multidisciplinary teams
- Support of carers

However, it would be hoped that this approach to assessment and care will become normal for all patients – especially, but not exclusively, those with long-term progressive diseases. Health care should aim to support patients and their families to make appropriate decisions, plan for the future, and cope with the symptoms and issues that arise. All professionals involved need to provide integrated, collaborative, and coordinated care for their patients so that their quality of life is as good as possible and to support their families and carers throughout their illness and into bereavement.

We should all aim to provide care, compassion, empathy, and justice [4] for our patients, their families, and ourselves, as professionals.

References

1. National End of Life Care Programme. End of life care in long term neurological conditions – a framework for implementation. http://www.endoflifecareforadults.nhs.uk/assets/downloads/neurology_report_final_20101108_1.pdf. Accessed 17 Apr 2012.

2. EAPC. People with neurological disease. 2012. http://www.eapcnet.eu/Themes/Specificgroups/
   Peoplewithneurologicaldisease/Guidelinescurriculumtaskforce.aspx. Accessed 17 Apr 2012.
3. National Institute of Clinical Excellence. NICE Clinical Guideline 105: motor neurone disease;
   the use of non-invasive ventilation in the management of motor neurone disease. London:
   National Institute of Clinical Excellence, London; 2010.
4. Hanks G, Cherny NI, Portenoy RK. Introduction to the fourth edition: facing the challenges of
   continuity and change. In: Hanks G, Cherny NI, Christakis NA, Fallon M, Kaasa S, Portenoy
   RK, editors. Oxford textbook of palliative medicine. 4th ed. Oxford: Oxford University Press;
   2010. p. 1–2.

Index

D. Oliver (ed.), *End of Life Care in Neurological Disease*,
DOI 10.1007/978-0-85729-682-5, © Springer-Verlag London 2013